ENDORSEMENT

Written by an ER nurse of 20 years, these real life stories give an entertaining sample of what goes on in the ER on a daily basis. Although concise, each story has a nice balance of medical accuracy and character that is easy to follow for those readers who have never worked in the medical field. Because the stories are told from a personal perspective rather than focusing on medical jargon, the reader sees the ER from a softer side where some important and often funny life lessons come to life.

There is plenty of entertainment for everyone with each chapter containing excitement, comedy, and heart-warming scenarios; this book makes a great conversation piece for any household. Once the reader experiences one story there is a desire to read more and move onto the next case as there is always something new ahead.

I hope you enjoy this book as much as I did.
Cassandra L. Ashley, M.D.

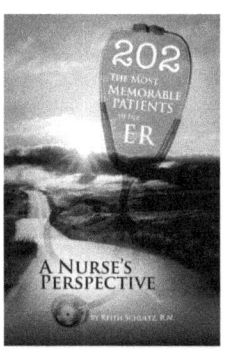

Cover by Kandace Schultz:
Road to the Sunset of a Memorable Career in ER Medicine

—

202 MOST

MEMORABLE

PATIENTS

IN THE

ER

A NURSE'S PERSPECTIVE

by Keith Schultz RN

Printed in the United States of America
ISBN: 978-1490504582

—

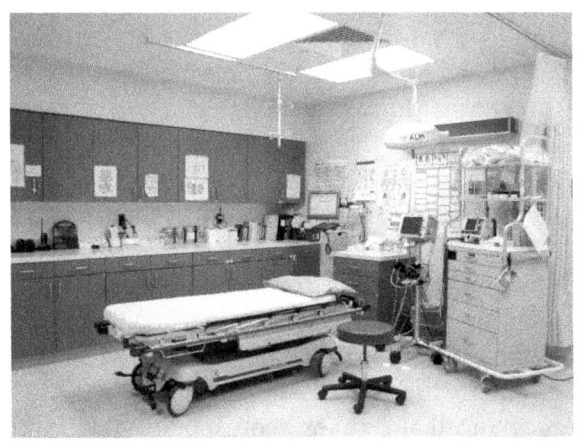

Preface

Events that made this book possible

In the process of writing this book there were more memories flooding my mind than those that were recorded. These included the co-workers that will be family forever, every square inch of the halls and rooms; the supply rooms where I could find supplies blindfolded if necessary; and how each room had a special meaning. There wasn't enough room to write everything about the emergency department that was a part of my career, but at least I was able to record some of it here.

Many times my patients would ask how I got into the health field and why. If their prognosis was good I had a stock story of facts with a twist. I would say, 'I graduated from college with a degree in forestry at the height of the Dutch Elm Disease epidemic. It was my job to aggressively treat the elm trees to save them, but most died. Next I bought a Western Auto Store fixing tires, changing spark plugs, replacing batteries but all eventually died, and were junked.

So I thought I would try humans for a while!" Reactions were unanimously the same; laughter, and then wondering if they should get another nurse. But most would always want me to continue, even more then before.

—

My daughter is completing her RN training this August 2013. She is following in my footsteps getting her start in nursing late in life. I am proud of her for accomplishing the same goals I did, while raising a family with her husband's support and a teenage son.

My son is also in the health field as a research specialist, finding ways to better take care of patients for Stryker Medical Corporation. Pride abounds as I watch him follow my love of health care.

I want to thank my wife for the sacrifices she made, and the support and encouragement she gave me so that I could pursue my ambitions and career changes to get to where I am today.

I also want to thank Cassandra Ashley, MD for editing the medical accuracy in all the cases represented and Kandace Schultz for the graphic designs.

Finally, I'd like to thank my editor, Diana Ross, for her contributions to the finalization of this book.

At least now, when I kick into a memory mode, I can pick up this book and quickly be transported to the "good old days".

****

—

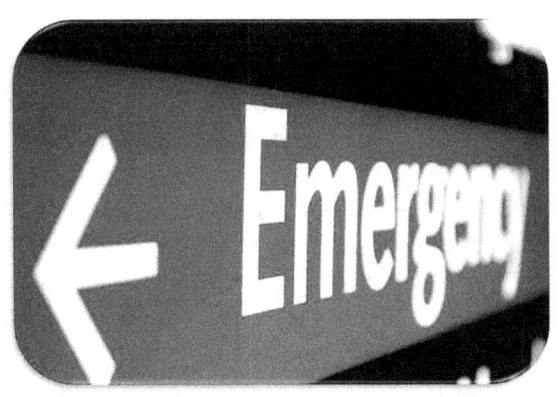

INTRODUCTION

What circumstances make an Emergency Room patient memorable? Of the hundreds of patients who are treated each day what makes one or two stand out the next day or even the next week? Does the kind of illness or trauma make the difference?

Is the answer in the way he or she dressed? Is it the type of reaction the patient had to the pain or illness? How about the way she or he walks? Whether obese, skinny, swelling, or blood covered, variables surrounding the cause of the ER visit can make that one patient of that one shift stand out more then any of the others.

There are not any recorded notes taken during the shift to help remember. Each case is simply written sitting down at home, thinking of the previous shift. Who, if any, stand out? When an image forms in the mind it is duly recorded, as to looks and presentation and history. Are the patient's actions consistent with the problem given? In other words, if she said her knee is injured is there a limp? If his belly hurt does he walk bent over in pain? It merely takes a "first impression" during the first few seconds of observation to figure out if this patient might become a memorable candidate.

Once in a while the patient or the injury is a good part of the memory but it could be the events leading up to the ER visit. Such things as how it happened, the means of getting to the ER or even the patient's history before the event adds the extra detail. Whatever that little thing that makes the patient memorable is never known until it is time to record that last shift.

How can one categorize the memorable patients into a book? Each chapter might be by gender but that results in only two chapters. How about age? That might be as many as 90 or more chapters. Let's try size. That doesn't work either.

The best way to present the most memorable patients is to have each chapter a different type of illness since that does not make any difference in determining how memorable he or she might be. The same arrogant, obese, loudmouth is as memorable with abdominal pain or an ingrown toenail. He is memorable whether his illness is critical or not. The quiet, well-dressed person with a polite voice is memorable with a deep laceration or a rash from an allergic reaction. It is the person not the illness; the reaction not the pain; the attitude not the thoughts; and probably more about a person's cultural background than the current problem.

There are 202 patients recorded in this book and are selected from over 2500 memorable patients recorded during portions of 20 years of Emergency Room nursing. Some fact or statistic about each patient is altered to protect the identity without taking away from the events that make them memorable. In some cases the appearance and clothes from one patient was used to describe another patient. These did not take away from the primary case but helped describe the actions and reactions.

Any resemblance to any living or dead person is purely coincidental. The actual person might be fat but presented slim. The person might be a female but really is a male. The age is different only to the point that the reality of the illness or injury is not altered. For instance, a person suffering from chronic arthritis could not be changed from an older person to a teenager and be realistic. The cases are real; the treatments are appropriate; and the outcomes are true.

TABLE OF CONTENTS

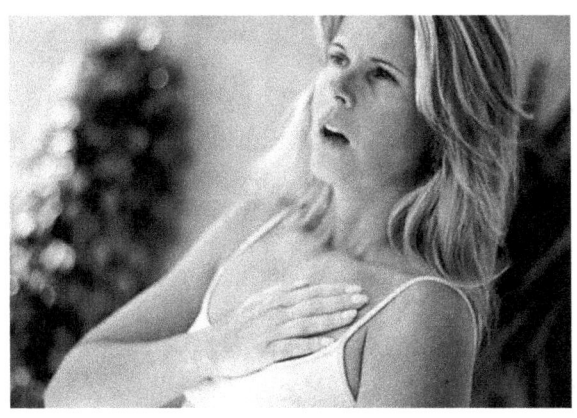

CHEST PAIN

When is "chest pain" considered a heart attack and when is it one of dozens of other causes? Most of the time those magic words, "chest pain" results in a rapid and full set of protocol procedures in the ER. It is not worth the consequences to do anything but react in a worse case scenario and to miss one heart attack. Many times "chest pains" are not a heart related problem. After ruling out a heart attack the patient would get a diagnosis for the real problem and be treated accordingly. Below are some examples, and how they happened and the reactions.

****

A young single gal of 38 came in with chest pain for the third time in 2 weeks. Each of the other two times all tests were negative for heart problems and she was sent home with pain medications. Was this visit just to get more pain pills or was the pain real? The way she presented herself, apologizing, with a voice that seemed to quiver with fear, most of the staff believed she was in real pain. She was not obese and appeared to be in relatively good physical condition.

Her history included a lot of stress in the recent past. Both parents had not been in good health and had lived with her. Eight months ago, she found her father dead in his bed when he did not come to breakfast. Two weeks ago she had found her mother dead on the kitchen floor with a heart attack. Crying daily was a normal occurrence the past few weeks.

Stress might affect the human body in strange ways like chest pain, indigestion, headaches, and more. This quiet and patient gal was willing to repeat all previous tests and more. The normal tests for a cause of the pain did not reveal anything.

Finally the radiologist report came back indicating the presence of a blood clot in the left lung. What a relief. Everyone wanted a diagnosis for her pain and illness. She cried with joy over the bad/good news.

She was admitted with IV blood thinners for a few days. At discharge her thank-you visit to the ER was welcomed. She cried again but this time it was from appreciation.

****

A 54 year-old man came in saying he had "chest tightness". The symptoms started that night while he was in the kitchen cooking a meal. Chest tightness was the key phrase for getting a protocol workup for heart problems even though he had no other symptoms that went along with a heart attack. Three hours later all tests were back showing the heart was not a part of the tightness feeling. Since no "chest tightness" diagnosis was made in the ER he was admitted for further tests such as stress test, ultrasound, gastric, and more. Most patients were not admitted for the symptoms he presented but he was the exception, which made this patient worth recording.

He was a Vietnam Veteran. Most of his platoon had been lost in a grenade explosion that burst both of his eardrums and required him to wear hearing aids. Later, he lost his left leg below the knee from gunfire, plus a napalm fire caught him in a back draft putting him in a coma for months. The VA hospital prescribed him numerous sedative drugs for bedtime to control nightmares. He wore a prosthesis on his lower leg. He had never had any cardiac problems but a doctor cannot disregard a person's past and current history.

Each staff member took time to say 'thank-you' and 'good luck". He was still active in the VFW and that was where he had been cooking for the troops during their bingo night.

****

In the middle of the night a 50 year-old man came in complaining of "chest pressure". An EKG tracing of the heart did indicate possible early onset of a heart attack. Immediately all the IV meds and pills were given to this patient of average height and weight.

Following by-pass heart surgery one year ago he had a stroke that affected his left side. Rehabilitation got those limbs to work well, but his face had some residual drooping. He was quiet spoken with no panic or even concern about the possible diagnosis.

That day he had been helping his newly married son move some furniture, but denied lifting anything heavy. He denied any chest pain in the afternoon, but in the evening hours he would stand upright with a little "chest pressure". Bending forward at the waist increased the pressure that radiated into both sides of the neck. Straightening back to an upright position the pressure would almost go away. This symptom history was inconsistent for a person with a heart problem.

After a cardiologist consult the diagnosis did not include a heart attack. He was having muscle strain of the muscles in his chest, from lifting too much that day. It was his wife's turn to become verbal and remind him that all day she kept telling him "not to overdo it." His reply, "Yes, dear."

****

A 53 year-old woman complaining of chest pain was brought into the ER by a deputy from the jail. This was a common inmate ploy just to get out for a while and possibly be admitted. Earlier that day, she had been driving in an erratic manner, and fled the deputy sheriff by speeding to her home.

She was not cooperative and resisted arrest. She looked many years older because her face had deep furrows from years of a tough life. She had a potbelly from her excess drinking and lack of taking care of herself. A complaint of chest pain on the scene resulted in an ambulance being called. She would not let them treat her, so she was taken directly to jail.

Later she became uncontrollable and was sprayed with pepper spray. The 'chest pains' returned and that was when she was brought to the ER. She remained uncooperative with verbal abuse to all and profanity more the kind from a man. She refused any kind of vital signs to be taken or any other heart attack protocol. When she became increasingly more combative she was restrained with wrist and ankle restraints. This allowed an EKG to be performed, which was normal. She was discharged to return to jail. The continued excess profanity could be heard out to the parking lot.

****

A 63 year-old male came into the ER complaining of sharp chest pain, not a typical heart related type of pain. It had progressively started while watching TV, and 2 hours later it was worse, with difficulty breathing. All the chest pain protocol orders were activated.

He was obese and worked at a desk with no outside activities. There was no cardiac history including relatives. He stated he'd had a cold the past week. Lung sounds and x-rays did show slight pneumonia in both lungs. The diagnosis did not go far enough. Certain test findings confirmed the symptoms presented by a patient and further tests were canceled. The patient was sent home with some antibiotics.

The following night he came back saying not only did he have the sharp pains with each breath, it also felt like an anvil was sitting on his chest. Along with sweats and reports of vomiting prior to arrival he was put on the fast track for heart attack protocol testing.

Shortly he ended up in the cath lab where they found a 95% blocked artery. Therefore, all these so called "chest pains" need to get a full workup every time. He came in apologizing for coming back so soon, but it was the ER team who apologized in the end.

****

A nursing home called to say they were sending in a person with chest pain. It was a 60 year-old man that confessed to weighing 400 pounds, but could have weighed more. During the assessment in ER, he stated that he kept complaining to the nurses at the nursing home of a burning pain like a "hot poker" starting in his feet and going up all the way to his head. This resulted in a headache. He self-diagnosed himself as having a stroke but was told strokes do not have pain like that. After his other complaints did not work this resourceful man came up with "chest pain". Those words got him the action he had been looking for all day. The ambulance was called to transport.

He was a whining person with all kinds of things wrong with him and said he never got any help with his main complaint, that burning pain. Since he was brought in for chest pain, all the tests were being completed. In the meantime it was explained that his diabetes was causing neuropathy, which is a burning sensation. If he lost a lot of weight the burning sensation would probably be less. All heart related tests were negative. His blood sugar was 260 so a shot of insulin was administered.

When he was discharged to go back to the nursing home his brother came to the ER in a VW bug – way to small for the patient's bulk. The ambulance had to be called to take him back. Most of the staff wondered if the brother had done that on purpose to avoid the whining he knew was going to happen the entire trip back.

****

The husband of a 54 year-old lady came running into the triage area yelling, "Help, help - my wife is having a heart attack - she is a nurse and knows what she is talking about". The first symptom she mentioned was a sharp pain in the right side. Since most heart attacks are pressure pains and on the left side, the validity of the nurse's diagnosis was in question.

Per proper protocol, the tests were administered. The doctor's diagnosis was "Atypical chest pain" meaning a muscle strain or bruise. She went home pain-free after the medication was properly given for the diagnosis. The patient's nursing background was nurse aide in a nursing home.

****

A nurse working in the cardiac care unit of the hospital had a patient recovering from bypass heart surgery. This 36 year-old gal was very good at her job dealing with heart patients. But when it came to her own "chest pain" she failed the test miserably of which she admitted freely in the days that followed.

She mentioned to her charge nurse about the chest pain she

had been experiencing the past 20 hours. She was sent to ER for a work up. Her request was to have a blood draw and then go back to work. If the results indicated she was having a heart attack she would come back. She was informed it definitely did not work that way. She was here to stay until all tests were back.

Her primary symptom was a pinpoint sharp pain on the upper part of her left chest. No other symptoms such as sweats, nausea, shortness of breath, or weakness. It did not get worse coming down the steps or walking. In other words, she was a cardiac nurse but did not know the symptoms of a heart attack. She only knew the results after the heart attack was corrected. It was not a mark against her, but a lack of experience. All nurses in that department have to pass an ACLS course – Advanced Cardiac Life Support. She had either not taken the course or had forgotten what it taught.

Three hours later, it was determined that it was either nerve pain or a pulled muscle. She was discharged to return to her unit for work. She got a good education in the ER and will now be a better unit nurse.

****

A 28 year-old obese male came waddling into the ER hyperventilating about 60 breaths per minute. As a result his hands were curling inward making a fist with white knuckles. His skin was pale and his stride was unbalanced. He appeared about to fall due to dizziness. When a word could be spoken between breaths it was about chest pain. He gasped it hurt so bad he wanted to die.

His chest was palpated to find the spot that hurt the most, and when it was found he screamed in pain. There was no specific spot but a small area was extremely sensitive. His hyperventilation continued unabated.

An IV was started after forcefully uncurling his arm. The magic medicine, an anti-anxiety drug, was given to calm things down so a cause of the chest pain could be determined. Gradually the breathing slowed and the chest pain disappeared. His curled arms and hands were able to straighten with help. His medical history was void of hyperventilation and chest pain. He had recently gotten a divorce and lost his job. Stress can do crazy things to the human body.

****

6

A hospital employee brought in a 77 year-old neighbor having chest pain with a recent history of a heart disease. A few weeks ago she had an angiogram with findings of multiple blocked arteries of the heart. She refused to have bypass surgery and was convinced she would either heal or die – whatever the Lord wanted.

Thorough tests were conducted showing no changes. Also there were no new indicators of a heart attack. Because of her past history she would be admitted, but the consensus was that she would check out against medical advice. She made it clear she would refuse any angiogram or operation.

While being transported upstairs she told new events in her life she had not revealed earlier. She was in the process of moving 100 miles from her hometown, the third most stressful event in a person's life. She felt anxious about finding new friends even though her daughter lived there. She may have been elderly and stubborn, but was soft spoken and carried a big stick. She admitted the stress was almost too much to bear.

FYI – the number 1 and 2 stressors in a person's life were reported to be marriage and divorce. Some have said "death" is really number 1 – but who could prove that?

****

A 44 year-old female was complaining of "chest pain". No amount of tests would confirm a case of heart attack. When asked about the medications she took on a regular basis, she produced a long list. Two antidepressant meds and a nerve pill were included. When asked if she was diagnosed with depression the reply was a strong "No". Since she also had a nerve pill the question became whether she was bi-polar or more correctly, manic-depressive. Again there was a strong negative response. The consensus was she was either embarrassed to admit it or in denial.

She walked and sat in a slouched position with head hanging low and would not look anyone in the eye. All movements were on the slow side like calculated thoughts of each action. Rumbled hair that hung heavy onto her shoulders appeared to not have had a good shampoo in a long time. The monotone of her voice was the most distinctive part of the impressions by the staff.

During the 3 hours of testing she did at one point show a slight manic state but quickly returned to a quiet state. Something was going wrong, and to be safe she was admitted to the hospital with a diagnosis of "chest pain". How unique.

****

A 66 year-old lady came in complaining of chest pain after vomiting numerous times brought on by "bad food" earlier. She had quite a large belly sticking out below the ribs, as if she had swallowed a watermelon. When asked if she had bloating problems she became upset. Seems she was sensitive about her fat tummy. An explanation of concern about combined vomiting and bloating may be important to know. She re-emphasized the chest pain.

When asked about the exact location of the pain she pointed with a finger to the bottom end of the breastbone. She said it was a sharp, burning pain. The suspect diagnosis indicated she was having inflammation of the esophagus from the acid in the vomit. However, the "chest pain" protocol occupied 3 hours of her time.

A special drink containing a numbing medicine for the entire upper gastric system gave her complete relief long before the heart tests were completed. She thought it was a miracle drug and wanted a prescription for it. She was amazed that the right things were done so quickly. She also understood more about chest pains as opposed to stomach pains.

****

She was 34 years old, single, not very good-looking and possibly in search of attention. In the past 3 months her ER visits included a sore back, cough, fever, hurt leg, and twice with chest pains. Each time she insisted she needed to be admitted for pain control. This visit was another "chest pain" along her left side rated at a 10 out of a 1 to 10 pain scale. That means by definition, the worst pain she had ever experienced in her life.

While lying on the cot her arms circled her chest in a self-hug position. When the chest was palpated during assessment she would yelp with pain saying that made it worse.

People like this got little empathy from the ER staff. She again had negative results for all possible pain sources for her symptoms. An over-the-counter pill was offered but refused and she was discharged. Probably tomorrow night she will be back for another attempt at getting admitted. Should the staff have been more sympathetic for a person who felt compelled to live like that?

****

A car came screeching into the ambulance bay. The driver ran through the doors with panic in her voice, saying her husband was dying of a heart attack. She said she had driven 16 miles in 20 minutes on mountain roads to get here. The man, clutching his upper abdomen with an open hand, was put into a wheelchair and transferred to the trauma room. Quickly respiratory techs, x-ray techs, nurses, EKG techs and a doctor appeared, doing their tasks in the chest pain protocol.

The 44 year-old was writhing and moaning, making it difficult to start the IV, apply the oxygen, and take a chest x-ray. Regardless, within 10 minutes the results of the heart tracing was complete and all other protocol tasks were completed. After all the results were back the diagnosis was, "a normal, healthy heart."

The doctor announced the results to the patient and his wife. Immediately the patient stopped the loud moaning, and the fear of pending doom in his eyes was no longer apparent. His arms relaxed, the shoulders slumped, leaving only the soft moans of pain like a whimper. The wife had the same reaction with tears slowly drifting down her cheeks. All techs and extra staff left the room.

The patient was told he would have to drink a bad tasting slurry (nicknamed by one of the doctors as "the green lizard") to get rid of the pain. He said, "Bring it on." The diagnosis was stomach acid burped into the esophagus causing a severe burning irritation – commonly called 'heartburn'. Within 3 minutes of drinking the medicine the pain was gone and it was quiet in the room, except for the muffled sobs from the wife as she released the tensions within.

****

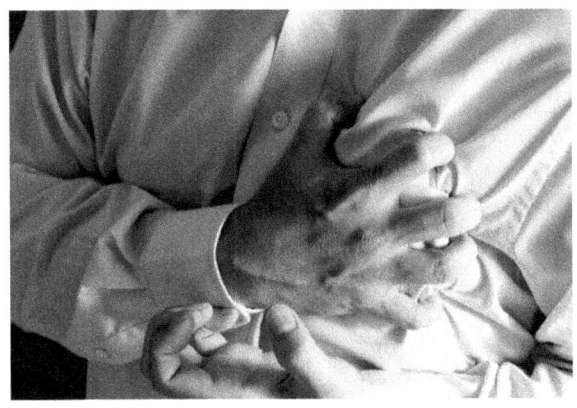

<u>HEART</u>

Treating heart attacks becomes a norm in the ER to the degree that every nurse learns the protocol well, since it happens one or more times nearly every shift. The patient makes the difference in each case. Some may come in scared of possible death and others are accepting of the possible outcome or at least have faith in the caretakers to save his life. Differentiating the kinds of "heart attacks" is the challenge. The patient can be so calm the diagnosis becomes a matter of reading the signs more than the symptoms he or she expresses. Others scream in eye-popping fear and the worry exaggerates the actual condition.

****

A lady calmly walked through the ambulance doors to the ER stating she was having "heart palpitations", and needed "that drug that stops the heart" so it would correct her funny feelings. This eerily calm and systematic 52 year old asked which room she should go into for treatment. She was already unbuttoning her blouse when she got to the room. Without any instructions from the staff, she undressed to the waist and promptly was lying on the cot. Everyone was in shock because of her calm and systematic actions and even temperament.

She proceeded to give her medical history, which included at least a dozen times that this had happened to her. Each time an IV was started and a drug was given that "stops my heart and corrects the problem, when it starts going again."

The whole staff was well aware of everything she was referring to about her condition and treatment. The "shocking" part was the reference to "stopping the heart" was usually never discussed with the patient, only between medical staff. Most people would not even want to know about a drug that "stops the heart". The usual statement was a "drug that corrects the heart beat."

Since this lady had been through this procedure many times, she was almost begging to get on with it. The doctor gave the order and it was given. She did not twitch an eyelid as the monitor went crazy, and then revealed a straight line followed by a pause, meaning the heart had stopped. After a few big blips on the monitor the wonderful normal waveforms appeared. She smiled and said "Thank-you" while sitting up requesting all leads and IV be disconnected, so she could go home. That request did not get realized immediately, because all the treatment protocol completed on her happened so fast no documentation had been completed; such as her name, age and other pertinent information. After an observation period of 2 hours she was discharged. Sure was an easy case.

****

"Just a little pressure feeling in the middle of my chest", was the only complaint a slim, smiling 72 year-old woman made when she walked into the ER triage. She also stated her heart was "vibrating" making it feel like her whole body was shaking. Those words were ominous keys to take action with a wheelchair ride into the nearest trauma room. Quickly, she was undressed to allow for an EKG and other protocol to be completed.

A quick manual pulse check indicated a rate of 160 beats per minute. She denied any nausea or sweats as the ER technician attached the leads to her chest for an EKG, as more questions were asked. The patient looked as if she were going into shock while quietly lying on the cot. Later she admitted everything since her arrival had happened so fast she "sort of froze" with anxiety. "It was the first time in my life I was rushed to a room and two men stripped me to the waist and laid me on a bed" she said with a teasing smile.

Finally the monitor came on and did show a rate of 170 irregular beats per minute. She added other symptoms of weakness, dizziness, and of course the pressure in the middle of her chest. It was about a five-minute wait for the doctor and in that time she suddenly said, "Hey, I feel great. What did you do to me?"

When the doctor arrived the monitor indicated a rate of 84 beats per minute. He stated out loud that the patient was not really sick, but when the technician produced the print out of the EKG it proved different. He went to the patient who indicated no more weak feeling, or dizziness, or any pressure on her chest. In other words, she had converted to normal sinus rhythm while lying on the cot, before any intervention could be done. The lady was admitted to the cardiac unit for observation and more tests. Her only comment was, "Do I have to go through all this every time I want to be molested?"

****

The ambulance crew radioed the ER they were in route with an 86 year-old woman having a heart attack, and they were sending a full 12 lead EKG. The cardiologist and the cath lab crew were called, arriving before the ambulance, since it had been a long trip through lots of hills and curves to get to the ER. When the ambulance pulled in, everyone was waiting for the doors to open and a cot to appear. Instead, the rear ambulance doors flew open, followed by an announcement of a full code blue. Her heart had stopped just as they pulled into the ambulance bay.

A nurse was straddling the patient performing chest compressions as the cot was rushed to the trauma room. Then, suddenly a shout was heard, "Stop that, it hurts!" The patient was awake with regular pulse, good blood pressure, and was breathing. A quick apology was given as the nurse dismounted from the cot. Not realizing the importance of the chest compressions the patient continued, "What in the world were you trying to do to me? You made it hurt more than before and you're supposed to make it better, not worse!" In the few minutes she was in the ER, she never stopped complaining of "that nurse that made me feel worse."

Within 15 minutes she was in the cath lab and a major artery was opened, but more work was needed. A full heart surgery was done within 4 hours, followed by a touch- and- go prognosis for the next few hours.

This woman was tough, making a full recovery within the

next few days. Her friends reported she was smiling bigger than ever. Her only complaint was the rib pain in the middle of her chest. She was reminded that if it were not for the necessary inflicted pain she might not be here now, because it had saved her life. After a pause to contemplate this, her smile grew even bigger.

****

His go-cart at the local amusement park crashed. He got out of the cart and fell to the track. Personnel were quick to call the ambulance, but this 5 foot 8 inch, 250-pound man insisted he was ok. He said it was "only some pressure feeling on my chest." On arrival, the paramedics said he was sweating profusely and had nausea.

This information was radioed to the ER and the cath lab was alerted. The pain level of his "pressure" was moderate and described like "the go-cart had landed on me." He was classed as having an acute MI and would quickly be stabilized in the ER and transferred to the cath lab. The actual time from ER door to the cath lab was only 20 minutes.

The angioplasty was performed, opening 3 arteries. In recovery, he had nothing but praise for all the people involved at the racetrack that insisted he go to the hospital. He was only 49 years old and was now convinced to lose his extra weight and get heart healthy. He was discharged 2 days later to return home, some distance to the south, and follow up with a cardiologist, nutritionist and fitness trainer. Let's hope he keeps his promises.

****

A 68 year-old lady from the East Coast was staying in a motel while on vacation. In a scared, quivering voice that indicated a realization that this was serious, she related the events leading to her ER visit. She had shortness of breath on and off the past 3 days, especially during the night. She would wake up in severe breathing distress, but sitting up on the edge of the bed it would gradually get better. This caused more tiredness and she would fall backward, asleep, only to awaken a short time later in respiratory distress again.

A stethoscope to listen to her breathing indicated she had fluid in her lungs with possible pneumonia, caused by a less then efficient heart called congestive heart failure. When she heard the diagnosis her demeanor became surprisingly calm, with a wry smile and a smooth coherent voice. Her explanation was, "Wow, I thought I was about to die." When told she just might die if it were not corrected, she again changed completely to a worried, incessant-talking mass of worry. "Does that mean I am going to die for sure?"

When she was assured of survival with the help of the staff and being able to live a long time, she became calm once more. "You should not ever have told me that I could die. I thought it was going to be true." She did become calm and was discharged a few days later.

****

Each breath taken by an elderly patient created rattles deep down that could be heard across the room. Each inhalation was a forced gasp followed by a loud moan of blowing the air out on exhalation. The nurses and techs were busy getting the patient undressed and hooked up to the monitor, starting the IV, applying oxygen, and all other protocol procedures.

The doctor arrived in the room with the conversation sort of one sided. Question: "Are you short of breath?" Patient: "I (gasp) can (gasp, gasp) not (gasp) breathe." Question: "When did this start?" Patient: "Can't (gasp) breathe" (gasp, gasp). "Help me". The doctor wisely decided to quit the questions and ordered blood work and a CPAP, a breathing mask that delivers oxygen under pressure to force the fluids out of the lungs, back into the blood stream. This was followed by proper medications.

Over the next few hours this pleasant 76 year-old lady's breathing improved and she could talk with only a few stops per sentence to catch her breath. Later, she requested the need to go to the bathroom for "everything". Since different machines were attached to her, a bedpan was provided. It was not known "everything" included explosive diarrhea that got her, the sheets, and the bed quite dirty. By the time the cleaning of her and the bed were done, her adrenalin from embarrassment helped get rid of most of the fluid in her lungs. The repeated ring of, "I'm sorry, I'm sorry" proved she could breathe better without the sound of Niagara Falls.

She was cooperative and pleasant during the entire time in the ER and was admitted to CCU for congestive heart failure.

It was the middle of the night when a 68 year-old man came walking into the ER complaining of severe left flank (side) pain with off and on nausea the past few days. He was placed in a room with oxygen applied and a pulse oximeter on his finger, indicating oxygen saturation of 97% and a pulse of 68. No heart monitor was used for the symptoms presented, as they indicated a possible kidney stone. An IV was started with pain medications that worked well.

The doctor's assessment agreed the symptoms did warrant a kidney stone cat scan, which confirmed all suspicions. Shortly after returning from the cat scan it was noticed the oxygen saturation was now 93% and the pulse was 40. The heart monitor leads were applied, and confirmed a dangerously slow heart rate.

The patient was nauseated, stating this was how he felt a few times earlier in the week. There was also a scared look in his eyes as the heart rate got slower and slower. The doctor was informed of the changes.

The diagnosis was "sick sinus syndrome", the failing of the part of the heart that generates the start of every heartbeat. He was told a cardiologist was his next doctor, before the urologist would be able to deal with the kidney stone. Besides being grateful to the ER for finding the heart problem, he was indebted to the kidney stone for bringing him. His analysis of the night was, "It must have been destiny that made all this happen the way it did."

****

If a man ever owed his life to his wife, it was a 70 year old brought into the ER via ambulance. He had not been "feeling good" for over 48 hours beginning with a shortness of breath after little exertion. He weighed over 300 pounds, meaning it did not take much to "exert". He denied any sort of chest pain, nausea, or sweats. The wife had been encouraging him to see the doctor from the very beginning.

Sitting quietly watching TV he gradually had increasing difficulty breathing without any exertion. That was when his wife stopped urging and called the ambulance. He first agreed to allow them to just check him out. Of course that meant a trip to the ER with lights and siren, when the monitor showed a pulse of over 230 beats per minute. In route, they called the report in, adding history of "Agent Orange Induced Diabetes" as a Vietnam Veteran. It did not include any heart disease, or even high blood pressure as so many obese people have.

The doctor gave the paramedics orders to treat the current condition. On arrival to the ER 45 minutes later, a jolly man with a tummy like Santa was laughing and joking. His wife reported the change in personality from happy, to silent and somber, in the past 48 hours and now back to jolly was amazing. He admitted, "I am a stupid, stubborn, old man that should listen to my wife of 44 years." His wife just smiled and I am sure recorded that statement to long-term memory.

He was a very lucky man to endure a dangerous heart condition for an indefinite amount of time that could have killed him. There was not a moment of hesitation on the part of the patient or his wife when he was told he was to be admitted for further cardiac tests and more.

****

With the appearance of impending doom in his eyes, the 69 year-old man uttered in a scared, high-pitched whine, "Please, don't let me die". He was on a cot in a trauma room, having been brought by private car to the ER. He was having severe chest pressure, profuse sweating, and had vomited prior to arrival. These were a true set of emergency signs and symptoms that needed fast assessment and care. The patient's attitude at the moment would work against his outcome.

The nurse in charge of his care immediately explained to him that any person able to talk on arrival while having a heart attack had never died in this ER room while under his care. The nurse added that a few years ago he was the person lying on this same cot having a heart attack. He said he was living proof of a full life after such a crisis.

Immediately the patient let his shoulders slump, the clenching of his jaws relaxed, and the eyes lost that look of doom. The next request was, "Then take this pain away." Pain meds and heart meds helped very little.. He insisted he hear again the details of the nurse's experience and what it took for him to get pain relief. He all but called the nurse a liar.

The cath lab team took this big man away shortly, as he stared back toward the crew he was leaving. Assurances from the nurse pushing his cart were heard as he disappeared down the hall.

A few days later, this muscular man with a now normal deep, raspy voice came into the ER after his discharge from the cardiac unit. He wanted everyone to know how much he appreciated them. He then said, "The best thing was the reassurances I got from the nurse who said I was not going to die, and he was proof."

****

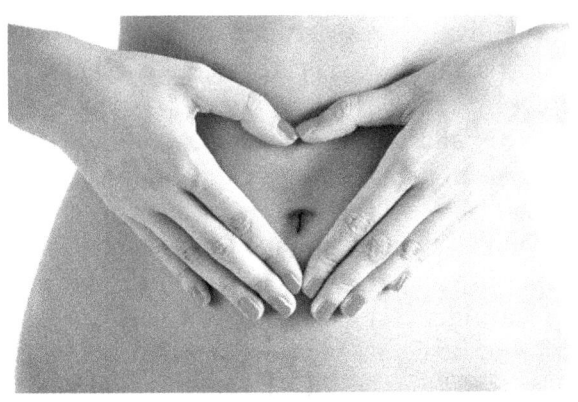

ABDOMEN

Abdominal pain is one of the most common medical complaints in the ER. Most any nurse will say it accounts for at least 50% of the cases handled in a shift. An anatomy lesson will tell the story.

There is the stomach, the small intestines, the large intestines, the liver, the pancreas, the ovaries, the bladder, the uterus, the prostrate, and the kidneys shoved into a very small area called the "abdominal region". Also there is stool (poop) along the way.

Gallstones and kidney stones cause severe acute pains, while ulcers and different types of indigestion cause chronic pains. In other words, this is an area consisting of many organs that can get painful. Even adhesions from previous surgeries have to be considered. There are also those people who come in complaining of "chest pain" who will point to a source well within the abdominal region.

****

A slender 50 year-old lady was doing the "kidney stone dance" as she stumbled through the ER. She was moving her hips in every position, twisting, thrusting, and stretching while walking in jerky steps at the same time. The quick, sidestepping gait made keeping her balance difficult, resulting in bouncing off both walls of the hallway. A side pain that would not go away no matter what position the body was in caused the "dance". The patient kept repeating, "I can't make the pain go away, please help."

In her case, she had awakened with the pain in her left flank, where the 'love handles' are located, stating, "I have never experienced this much pain – even during childbirth. It feels like the kidney stone I had last year."

An IV and a small amount of medicine was all that was needed to accomplish a 'pain free' condition. A cat scan confirmed the presence of a kidney stone in her left ureter near the bladder, with a prediction of being able to pass shortly. She was given some strong pain pills to take as needed and sent back to her motel with assurances that the stone would pass within 24 hours. There still was stumbling and near bouncing off the walls at discharge but it was from the narcotic meds this time.

Her parting comment was, "If I am not doing the waltz by morning I will be back, that is a promise." She did not return.

****

Both the doctor and off-going nurse were suspicious when the family of a sweet 80 year-old lady wanted her to be admitted even though her condition was not serious. Their vacation would not be ruined if she were "babysat" by the hospital. On arrival her face did not show any distress, and she was lying comfortably on the ambulance cot. According to her daughter she had a "tummy ache, cough with fever, and chest pain". The first thing the patient clearly stated with no stutter or grimace was she did NOT have any chest pain – only some diarrhea but not any kind of pain.

Shortly a fresh assessment of the whole situation by the new nurse revealed some additional symptoms. A quiet sit down conversation pursued with the now smiling and amiable patient. 'Are you having any pain at all?' She denied any pain. Her daughter was sitting nearby and said, "Mother, be truthful and tell the nurse everything. Tell him about that pain you have had in the lower tummy".

The patient replied, "Oh, that pain – it's right here." She placed her hand in the lower right quadrant of her abdomen. 'How long have you had that pain?' "Oh, about 4 days." 'How bad is this pain?' - "Not too bad - but it's always there."

An explanation of the pain scale was given. If zero is no pain and 10 is the worst pain you have ever experienced in your life - what number is this pain you are having in your stomach? "Oh, I don't know - maybe an 8." That is a significant pain, considering most elderly people in this situation belittle the 'pain' issue.

Tests for a volvulus (twisting) of the bowel or some other type of partial obstruction came back showing that there was no twist of the bowel, but a significant enlargement of one part of the bowel (lots of stool) pushing the rest of the intestines over, causing a partial bowel obstruction.

She was admitted after making a notation to tell the previous shift doctor and nurse that this was NOT a case of "dumping". It was a case of the patient not wanting to "bother' the rest of the family during a vacation who had tried to suffer through it all.

The most important admit order given to the floor nurses that night was to give enemas until clear. Oh, what fun.

****

At 5AM, a 45 year-old female waddled in, doubled over complaining of "stomach" pain. She was holding her hand tightly against the right upper area of her rather plump abdomen near the gallbladder while talking in gasping breaths, since each breath made the pain worse. She looked "sick".

She was asked what she had to eat in the past 12 hours. The answer was slow in coming, "We had bar-b-cue ribs, and french-fries, with ice cream for dessert. About midnight we were watching a movie and had a pizza delivered." She awoke at 3AM with this extreme pain and some vomiting.

An injection for pain and nausea helped in less then a half hour so she could lie flat. A cat scan confirmed our suspicions. Surgery to remove the gallbladder was done later that day.

Upon discharge she was educated on a low fat diet. "Are you calling me "fat?" The nurse had a good reply, "This is not for your fat but for your pain." The patient accepted the reason with a knowing smile.

****

"I have been sick for the last 2 days", said a 77 year-old rather skinny male sporting a true "pot belly." The anxiety was apparent, along with pale colored skin wet from sweat, as the ambulance cot was wheeled into the ER. Other symptoms included weakness, dizziness, shortness of breath, and an occasional severe cramp in his lower abdomen. He denied any fever.

After the abdominal x-ray, his problem was revealed - stool impaction (official radiologist diagnosis – FOS = "full of stool".) A Fleets Enema produced some results but not nearly enough for relief. Due to his weakness and dizziness caused by forcing his bowel urges to eliminate, he was admitted. He did not know being "full of it" was a reason for being admitted to the hospital.

****

A 42 year-old overweight gal from "down south" with a pleasant southern drawl came into the ER with severe abdominal pain, bending over and assuming the fetal position on the bed. She was tender in the right upper quadrant of the abdomen, with pain radiating into her back. She was asked the 5 "F's," questions related to gallstones plus one more for good measure.
1. Are you "F"emale?
2. Are you "F"air? (Caucasian)
3. Are you "F"ertile? (still ovulating)
4. Are you "F"orty or more? (age - not waist or bosoms)
5. Are you "F"at? (overweight)
And just to be sure added the 6th "F".
6. Are you experiencing excess "F"latulence? (passing gas)
She had 5 out of the 6 risk factors. Orders included pain meds, nausea meds, and the ultrasound of the gallbladder. Surprisingly, the gallbladder was as good as new – nothing wrong. She, along with the several staff that was sure it was gallstones, kept saying why should there be a list of risk factors if it is not right.

She was diagnosed with gastroenteritis (inflammation of the intestine). The sweet gal from the south helped prove a lesson that tests were needed to rule out or confirm a diagnosis. And another lesson from her - not all women follow the rules.

****

A lady appearing to be in her late 40s came in complaining of a possible strained muscle in the lower back. Her hourglass figure caught the attention of everyone as she carried her head high with pride as best she could. She was a massage therapist who had started some new personal exercises. The "confession" as she called it, included that she had over- did them and then felt this strong pain near her side. The severe pain she described started in the left back and side (flank) radiating around to the left groin area. The pain also would get better from time to time and even go away – but muscles strains usually do not do that. Besides, she came into the ER doing a dance with jerking steps that did not stop.

The cat scan confirmed a 3mm kidney stone right at the opening of the bladder that should pass any moment. That moment came about 10 minutes later. She was given a filter funnel that caught the stone with her next visit to the bathroom. Problem solved, and the massage therapist would be able to continue her new exercises even at her true age of 64.

****

Four hours of bad smelling excrement plus having to clean up the bed and patient three times is not a good thing. This all started with a frail and underweight 92 year-old lady brought in by her son and daughter-in-law. They reported she had passed out on her home bedside commode and had vomited once en route, arriving with nausea and lower abdominal pain. Maybe she had a bowel obstruction. Maybe she strained muscles from cramping during the vomiting. Best way to find out was an x-ray.

It was ordered, but was not taken for 4 hours. Why? The abdominal pain suddenly became overwhelming with a rectal projectile explosion of ½ stool and ½ water. The smell was very bad. Cleaning her up, plus the bed, floor, walls and any other object in the line of fire took some time. After the episode, she felt a lot better with no pain. However, we weren't out of the woods yet. She had two more episodes, resulting in more cleaning, to a lesser degree because this time we were prepared. Four hours later x-rays confirmed an empty bowel.

The family left the room and waited outside the whole time, were grateful for all the "trouble" they had put us through but we kept assuring them that is part of our job. They were not there to see just how bad it had been, but this sweet little old lady explained to them in detail the "trouble" and extreme messes she had caused. The whole time, the family was trying to make her quit telling the gross details of her story.

****

A young - looking 60 year-old lady attired in expensive clothes was trying her best to look dignified when the ambulance brought her into the ER. It was a difficult chore since she was rating her pain level at a 9 and fast approaching a 10. She held her arms across the mid abdomen indicating the sharpness was centered near the belly button area. A generous dose of morphine resulted in a smile of gratitude progressing into a slurred speech that tickled everyone's funny bone. Soon there was quiet as the happy juice overtook the pain.

The x-ray did show a bowel obstruction in the form of a small twist probably caused by a muscle spasm that would not relax. The first order given after diagnosis was an NG tube. This is a small tube (but it appears the size of a garden hose when you are the patient) threaded into the nostril, down the throat, and extending to the far end of the stomach. It is an uncomfortable procedure. This proper lady was apprehensive even though she was drugged to the point of being high. "I know you said it has to be done but please is there any other way?" After much coaching she was a trooper and did not fight it at all.

****

A very large amount (750cc or ¾ quart) of fluid, bile, and acid was suctioned out through the tube from the stomach. The amount of pain relief was hard to determine since the morphine was still working. Even so, the conversation emitting from her mouth was constant and slurred and mostly unintelligible. It was the slow and twisted gestures of face and hands accompanying her words that made it a humorous sight to witness.

She was admitted and given a series of enemas along with continued suctioning through the NG tube. By the next day the pressure release from both ends allowed the twist in the bowel to become normal and she was then pain free without any morphine.

Her slurred words were gone and the memories of the past 12 hours were also gone. Too bad, she had been extremely entertaining.

****

A 79 year-old man came in with right lower abdominal pain. The symptoms led all of us to believe it was a possible appendicitis, but surely that could not be true in an older person like this. Perhaps it was 'urosepsis' - a bad infection of the bladder and urine. All efforts to get a urine sample failed. After drinking lots of water he was finally able to pee, and the urine was as clear as crystal. A cat scan of the abdomen revealed the original diagnosis of appendicitis.

The family insisted they wanted to leave, and drive back home to their own doctor and hospital about 200 miles away. They were warned that if it were appendicitis and it "ruptured" en route going home he would be a dead person before ANY hospital could be reached, so they decided to stay and have it taken care of.

****

The best of all screamers came from a wrinkled, tanned, tough - skinned older man on a bus tour. It had started in the evening with a sudden, sharp, lower abdominal pain near the left groin area. He said, 'It feels like I need to go to the bathroom REAL bad to either poop, or pass gas." His skin was cool, clammy, and so wet with sweat that tape would not stick. His blood pressure was so low it could not be taken in a normal manner.

Every time he had an attack, he would scream out in pain. He was given a lot of IV fluids but his blood pressure remained low. A medication for low blood pressure was added and more IV fluids helped enough to start the blood transfusion. The man's intermittent screams continued because we could only administer sparing amounts of morphine to prevent the blood pressure from dropping even more. Therefore a delicate balance had to be maintained.

A leaking aortic aneurism was the first concern. An ultrasound could not confirm an aneurism, due to the bulging bowels from stool and gas. Even so, it was serious and needed advanced care.

The surgeon was not available, meaning a helicopter transfer to a level II hospital was in his immediate future. As soon as his condition could be stabilized enough for the trip, the screams and our helpless feelings would leave with him.

The helicopter did lift off with our patient exactly 1 hour and 17 minutes after he came. The flight nurse reported later that a different type of narcotic given en route had helped the pain, and luckily did not drop the blood pressure.

A follow - up report told us his abdominal aneurism surgery used 22 units of blood products and he was now in ICU with blood pressures in the 90s. They repaired a 9 cm (very large) aneurism that was partially ruptured and leaking blood. His survival was in question. After a person needs large amounts of blood products over such a short period of time the odds were not good for a full recovery. Like a lot of ER cases, the final outcome would never be known.

****

The panicked face and high-pitched voice of a mother bringing her daughter into the quiet ER with the blanched, pale face of death was our next case. The reactions of the mother probably made the 16 year-old patient more terrified and fearful of dying. She arrived by ambulance from a local theater, having passed out while going to the bathroom. To be more precise, she was grunting and pushing, with the urge to eliminate. The mother was talking a thousand words per second and this increased when there was no ER room open, and her daughter was placed in the hallway on a cot. Convinced her precious girl was dying; she felt she needed to be put in a top-level trauma room to save her life. The staff was aware that the patient was breathing with eyes wide open and moving all limbs, all good signs.

The EMT report stated she was having severe pain in the left lower part of the abdomen. What causes pain there? Two principal organs reside in that section – the ovaries and the bowels. The girl was calming down and able to tell us she had not had any BMs for the past few days but was trying to go when she passed out. This is known as a vaso-vagal response via the vagus nerve being irritated by trying to force a BM. The mother was in shock by the bodily function language spoken to her "little girl". This 16 year old did not even know the term "bowel movement" but did know "poop".

Shortly a room became available and the nurse gave the girl a fleets enema and placed a bedside commode nearby. The mother was relieved that her sweetie was not going to die and the patient was relieved 2 ways – pain gone, and mother's look of panic gone.

****

A pleasant and plump (admitted to 240 pounds but looked heavier) 29 year-old gal arrived complaining of severe right lower abdominal pains. She was a good-looking gal after getting past the grimacing wrinkles from ear to ear caused by her moaning, and at times, muffled screams. At the end of 4 ½ hours all tests were negative, leaving a lot of wondering and pondering. The soft-spoken girl was very patient, and continually stated she also wanted to know the source of her pain and to keep trying even though the repeated pain meds were making her drowsy with sleep.

Being clueless of the diagnosis a review was presented to another doctor who suggested a possible kidney stone. Light bulbs started to shine all over the place when the patient suddenly remembered she had a right-side kidney stone a few years ago that felt the same. An x-ray study confirmed a large stone more then half way down to the bladder from the right kidney.

What normally would be a one-hour diagnostic procedure in this case took over 5 hours. But the patient was happy, and after 2 more hours of letting the drugs wear off, she could safely head home. Strong pain pills were prescribed with an order to follow up with the urologist. The overall lesson for the ER crew was to always keep an open mind from the beginning because the next patient might not be so accommodating.

****

She was 75 years old; weighing only 125 pounds with a protruding potbelly like a big beer drinker might develop. After lots of questions about pain, she admitted she had been having intermittent "bad" cramps. She insisted, "This big belly is not right but it just can't be the reason for all this dumb pain."

She was very sweet but her concern of her normally flat belly being oversized was her greatest concern. It took a little persuasion to get answers to personal questions like bowel movements and passing gas since that was a hush -hush subject matter in her conservative upbringing. Her bowel movements the past few days got a response of "normal". What was normal?

"Maybe 2 or 3 times the past week." Asked "how much each time?" (That was more personal then she was comfortable with, but after some patience she responded in a whisper, "Kind of watery and not much".

Suspicions of constipation and gas led to an x-ray that confirmed lots of stool and a whole bunch of gas behind it. The solution was explained in detail about using a fleets enema. This would facilitate the release of all that gas that was making the belly so big and painful. She asked with a menacing smile just above a whisper, "Does that mean I can let it rip with big farts?" Wow, what a shocking statement from this gentle and shy lady.

****

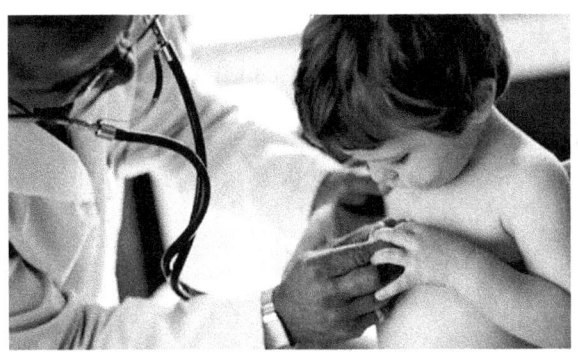

BABIES AND CHILDREN

Sick babies and children can be the most frustrating patients in the ER, but at the same time, the most rewarding. In a lot of cases they make fast recoveries using just an IV and fluid replacements. Dehydration quickly affects a child. They become listless, quiet and do not fuss or care what the procedure – to a limited degree. There are times a fever, vomiting, or diarrhea is present. Suppositories and other medicines can reverse the complications quickly, or they have to be admitted. Children and babies that are not as sick can be a challenge, not only to give medicine by mouth, but it can be a fight if an IV is needed. The following will help readers understand some of these complications that make them memorable.

****

A concerned neighbor saved a 20 month-old girl's life. The concern was an ongoing thing, because the mother frequently left her children alone for many hours at a time. At night she would go to parties, and would usually go shopping in the daytime.

It was mid afternoon when the neighbor heard strange sounds coming from the house and found a girl lying in the bed gasping for breath. This frail baby was using her accessory muscles in her stomach to breathe –called "retracted breathing pattern" meaning when a breath was taken, her stomach retracts excessively making her ribs stick out. It was a near respiratory failure situation and means the child was about as sick as can be and still be alive. The mother was not to be found in the house so the neighbor grabbed the child and rushed to the ER.

On arrival the pale, non-responsive baby had the look of death. Her hair was matted and dirty and she had very dry skin. Her lips were chapped, with dull mucous membranes inside the mouth – an ominous sign of advanced dehydration. Her feet and hands were black from dirt, with the exception of the finger on which she would eagerly suck.

She was put on high flow oxygen, an IV with fluid replacement going fast. Breathing treatments were begun, blood for labs was sent, and a chest x-ray ordered. She was diagnosed with pneumonia in both lungs, which would require intensive pediatric care. Transfer to another hospital was urgently needed. The baby was better at the moment but still considered critical. She looked like a rag doll, not moving her limbs or eyes.

Legally this initial treatment was done without parental permission to reverse the life-threatening situation. But once it was not quite as critical as before, the mother would now need to give permission for the baby to be transferred. The neighbor gave some clues as to where the mother shopped. The police located her at the supermarket. She was shocked her child was so sick, but had not been feeling good for about 2 days.

Police reported that the mother was about to start a prison sentence, unknown conviction, as soon as all her children were placed into foster care. Her sick baby would keep that from happening for quite a while. We wondered whether she had done this on purpose to keep from starting the jail sentence.

When the ambulance left to transfer the baby to another hospital, she was breathing better, resulting in a blood oxygen level of 88% rising to 92% only when she could muster a weak cry. A 96% would be considered low in a child.

The following day an update report from the pediatric intensive care unit stated she was no longer having retracted breathing and was maintaining a blood oxygen level of 95%. It was felt the neighbor who brought her into the ER should have gotten a medal of commendation. ER staff praised her.

****

A 3 year-old boy had been dropped off at his grandma's place 3 days ago. Grandma said it happened every time the boy got "sick" so his mother could go out and party. He had a low-grade fever and runny nose.

The past 3 days his fever had been up and down, reaching 103 degrees and only going down to 101 for about 2 hours after being given acetaminophen. He had not drank or eaten, and had not gone to "potty" when grandma decided he needed help in the ER. The underweight child just lay on the cot, content to just be quiet. No playing or restlessness,, or even looking around this strange and cold place called the ER.

His "quiet" was broken when the IV was started, but he did not fight like most boys his age. It was grandma and a tech that lightly held him still during the dirty deed. Before the lab results were back about ½ quart of replacement fluids were infused. What a change, in that hour. He was sitting up looking around asking all kinds of questions like "What is that?" "How does this work?" and more. Soon, he was able to drink water and was asking for something to eat.

He did have an upper respiratory infection and possibly a touch of pneumonia. Antibiotics were prescribed along with other appropriate instructions. Everyone got hugs from grandma and this precious boy had completely forgotten about that "dirty deed" and waved goodbye all the way to the door.

****

An eight month old learned very fast that a person wearing scrubs represented terrible things. She had a rapid heart rate of 160 per minute, breathing of 60 per minute with wheezing, a temp of 102 degrees and an eventual diagnosis of pneumonia and RSV. She was not spontaneously active and exhibited slight retracted breathing. Her parents were helpful and supportive of all procedures. The baby was not as helpful.

First, the IV made her cry and she kept trying to remove the needle from her arm, which meant applying a small board to that arm and lots of gauze and tape. Next was the test for RSV – a virus that lives in the upper part of each nasal passage. While holding her head still, a squirt of saline water went into the right nostril. This was the breaking point for the fast learning baby – her eyes were angry and the scowl was from ear to ear. The same procedure for the left nostril was done that added screams louder then before.

Next this baby was at her wits end when a small tube was shoved up to the back part of each nostril and suction applied to get a good wet sample.

The scowls, pouts, crying, and screaming continued after all the scrub attired staff left the room, leaving mother and father giving comfort. It took a while for her to calm down. She had learned that any person in scrubs was bad, and she would probably remember it for the rest of her life.

Next came the urine sample. A tiny bag that has an opening with sticky edges was applied around the genital area to catch the next urination. The screaming started at high decibels again.

Acetaminophen rectal suppositories created another trauma for her. A "breathing treatment" consisting of blowing a bad tasting medicine for the wheezing into her face so each breath would carry it to her lungs. She had plenty of deep breaths from her crying to make it work well.

From then on, even a person wearing scrubs who walked past the doorway meant the crying would start again. Soon this tired little "tortured" girl was sound asleep with a temp of less then 100 degrees and no wheezing. Breaths were 20 per minute and heart rate of 100 beats per minute. She was stable enough to be admitted to the hospital with more people in scrubs. Good luck to them.

****

A 5 year-old girl had an extensive medical history going back to her first year on this earth. At age 1 she was diagnosed with Cerebral Palsy; at 3 it was Autism; and just 1 year before, it was Epileptic Seizure Disorder. She did not walk or speak, and most of the time did not seem to understand what was said to her. There were temper tantrums, displayed by a hollering- type scream emitted in a low tone for such a young child, very loudly. These tantrums were heard in every corner of the ER.

Her night had started with a seizure at home that lasted over 7 minutes that ended with a period of quiet. Her doctor's orders had told her parents if a seizure lasted over 5 minutes, go to the ER. The ambulance was in route with her when another 2-minute seizure occurred. This time she came out of it with a "temper tantrum" hollering, kicking, and biting. The father was in the back of the ambulance to help. A few minutes later EMS reported she was calm and smiling and even a little playful.

When she was brought into the ER area, she had another temper tantrum while her dad tried to calm her down. According to her father, with so many visits to the hospital in her life she knew what could happen here and didn't like it. Another complication to her care was that she fought if anyone except her father and mother touched her. Needless to say, there was a lot of touching that had to be done. Restraining her for a rectal temperature, heart sounds, breathing and finally the blood draw was a 5 to 6 person procedure. Her parents insisted it was OK, as that was the only way it could be completed.

She needed a shot of medicine to calm her down but it was a long wait getting the order because the doctor wanted to wait for the lab results on her anti-seizure medicine blood levels. There were two more seizures and temper tantrums during that wait , disturbing all present including other patients and staff. Finally a shot of Ativan was given after another fight. When she was asleep peace reigned over all.

Her normal day was 3 to 4 seizures lasting from a few seconds to 3 or 4 minutes. It was suggested to discuss with her doctor about increasing the dose of seizure medication as the lab test indicated it was low. A lot of credit has to be given the parents. This unfortunate girl was still sleeping when discharged.

****

Ice cubes wrapped in a washcloth held to the lips of a 6 year-old girl usually means some kind of trauma has occurred. Her face did not have any blood on it and she was walking while softly crying. Another clue to the possible event was her stride – it was uneven that lead to a closer look for the pigeon-toed condition. The conclusion must be a fall striking her mouth.

The real story was she tripped over her own feet falling forward, meeting the corner of a magazine rack and hitting her mouth during the free-fall. She had a congenital defect in her hips that made her feet turn inward. This was being treated by Shriner's Hospital and she would eventually have an operation to correct it. Until then she fell frequently and was the reason mom and dad were not upset as it had happened too often in the past.

She had a small cut on the lower lip with bleeding under

control and a washed face before arrival. Dad had a baby tooth from the lower jaw in a zip lock bag. Her two incisors (the middle two upper teeth) were very loose. She was continually playing with these baby teeth with her tongue. The parents were hoping the missing tooth could be replaced and something done to stabilize the 2 incisor teeth.

It was recommended they not attempt to replace the tooth. The parents could not agree and called their own dentist who had the same answer as that given to them in the ER. No reinsertion needed, as a regular tooth will grow in there. Then he added a suggestion to remove the 2 incisors for the same reason, as they would not tighten up. Besides, the girl would continue to play with them until they fell out. The gaps created would last a little longer than normal, but would be better then having a tooth come loose and get caught in the throat or lung.

The incisors were removed with some screaming that sent the parents out the door. Then the 2 stitches in her lower lip went well, after soaking the cut with a numbing solution. She was scared, but with no pain during the first stitch she was an angel for the second stitch. All were happy at discharge, especially after the little girl was given a new stuffed animal from the ER stash of goodies.

****

A 19 month-old boy arrived in the arms of a worried looking mother explaining, "I think he may have taken one of my husband's heart pills".

"How do you know that?"

"Well, I turned around for just a second and heard this bottle spill on the floor. The baby was on the floor next to the spill and when I picked up all the pills there was one missing."

Most of the staff had many non-spoken questions to that story. First, if it was really a "second" of time" how could he have picked up a pill and put it in his mouth and swallowed? Most 19 month olds cannot take pills. Second, how did she know for sure that 30 pills were in the bottle? Third, how much of a search of the floor or open shoes or pants cuffs or other possible places was done to find it? There were no good answers to these questions, which meant the worst-case scenario must be assumed. Did the baby somehow swallow a pill for the first time in his short life, leaving no residue in his mouth from chewing?

The missing pill turned out to be an adult dose of a slow release beta-blocker which was considered an overdose if taken by a small child. Symptoms of overdose could include unusually fast or slow heartbeat, dizziness, slow or shallow breathing, seizures, unconsciousness, weakness, or fatigue.

The patient had been alert, talkative and playful since arrival. It had been less then an hour since the incident and a complete set of vital signs had been recorded. He kept indicating he did not "eat anything". He gladly drank some chocolate milk with activated charcoal. From then on, it was a waiting game.

Slow release beta-blockers reach a peak absorption in about 6 hours. This meant parents and staff would have to entertain the patient during this time and take another set of vital signs hourly.

Since it was late at night, it turned out he was a joy to have running around entertaining everyone instead of the reverse. He was happy, he was alert, he was a cutie and he never got tired. Plus, he was not sick. The staff played with him and his parents were a dream. The 6 hours went fast and they left relieved. They would probably find that pill lying in the middle of the room when they got back home. Then again it could be under a chair or it could never be found. All we knew was the child do not eat it.

****

A mother was awakened to the most terrible sounding cough she had ever heard from her 3 year-old son. It sounded exactly like the barking seals at the zoo. She called 911 when he started gasping and grunting, making a red face that turned blue from time to time. The ambulance arrived informing her this condition was called "croup" and must be reversed before it becomes "epiglottitis" which may swell the throat and block the airway.

On arrival to the ER a breathing treatment with the addition of racemic epinephrine and decadron had been prepared and was ready to blow into this child's face. The child was scared because all the action was coming at him so fast, but it was necessary to save his life. He was crying and twisting his head and turning in all directions to avoid the foggy mist being sprayed into his face. His mother held him in a big hug and a tech held his head. The crying was relentless, but for this kind of treatment the crying was good.

His actions forced him to take deep breaths to make the next cry, allowing the medicine to be pulled deep into his throat and lungs, enabling it to do the best job. He then tried to hold his mouth shut but could not breathe through his nose, and a sudden gasp of deep breath to catch up helped again.

The treatment was repeated once, taking 20 minutes before it was over and the hug from mother was released. Within 20 more minutes, the seal barking was gone and another 20 minutes his breathing was as normal as could be expected.

His crying and anger were quickly changed to smiles while he ate 2 popsicles with gusto and played with a gift of a coloring book, crayons, stickers, and even a stuffed Blues Clues. He was discharged with orders for mother, which included if this happened again, turn the shower on to hot and have the child breath the steam while waiting for the ambulance to arrive.

****

Two days ago a 14 year-old girl had her tonsils removed. Upon arrival in the ER she was holding her mouth wide open and breathing past the drooling since she had trouble swallowing. There was swelling in the throat with possible complications of a patent airway. She was more calm then her mother and was ready for anything to be done to help her. She had a hard time smiling because it hurt. A reminder was whispered in her ear that kissing boyfriends would have to be on hold for a while. Again, not even a hint of a smile, just a stare without any expression.

After the IV was completed and tape placed to secure it, she asked if it would hurt when the tape was taken off. "Yes, a little." She decided to take reciprocal action by taking a piece of tape and putting it on each staff member's arm. The promise was she got to "rip" off each of those pieces of tape when her tape was removed.

She was thirsty but did not want to drink anything. Therefore the IV fluids were rapidly infused while she was getting humidified air laced with special meds to reduce swelling. Soon she was breathing normally and able to swallow.

As she promised, when her tape was removed each staff member obediently held an arm out to have their tape removed. She really enjoyed the revenge – with a smile. Her one last act before leaving was a big kiss on the cheek for the nurse and the whispered comment, "You're wrong about the kissing."

****

One evening the sweetest little 3 year-old girl, who looked like Shirley Temple, came skipping into the ER. She had long curly blond hair, with a soft but penetrating voice. She was confused about all the excitement her parents exhibited about the drink she had thought was good. It was a sixteen-teaspoon dose of the grape flavored Dimetapp, a children's antihistamine. Her explanation was, "It's not medicine – it's grape juice." In high doses it will cause rapid heart rate with possible irregular heartbeats leading to possible fatality.

She thought all the patches placed on her chest for the heart monitor were cute stickers that could be pulled off and placed anywhere. She decided since they stuck so well and hurt to pull them off, she would just leave them. It was more fun to pull the snap off monitor leads and switch them around. Soon that was boring - thank goodness.

The second protocol for this drug was to drink activated charcoal that binds with all stomach and intestinal contents so absorption was lessened. This was mixed with chocolate milk, which this fun-filled girl was more then ready to drink. Part of the drink was a strong laxative. The parents were warned the first poop would be as black as activated charcoal.

For the next few hours during the slowest part of the night shift the whole staff played with the patient until she and her parents fell asleep. Mother slept on the cot with her daughter, and father went into a vacant room.

The monitor was watched closely. The high of 150 beats without any funny looking beats came at about 4 hours. These regular beats slowed down to 120 in the next hour. The parents were awakened for discharge. This beautiful little girl looked so innocent being carried out sound asleep.

****

Grandparents brought in a 7 year-old 'little lady' with a sore throat. She had a fever of 101 degrees plus a lot of pain when she swallowed, but she hated the drooling. She would force a swallow and then shake her head in disgust and open her mouth wide to breathe the cool air that soothed the throat. The smell of her breath was strong and distinctive of "strep throat". The throat swab was sent to lab for confirmation before medicine could be given. A liquid pain medicine was given in the meantime.

While waiting for the lab results the grandparents were asked how it came about this granddaughter was living with them. Immediately the girl, more mature then most, proudly proceeded to tell the whole story even though she had difficulty speaking past the sore throat.

"A long time ago (3 years) my mommy and daddy were killed in a car accident," she began. "I have 2 grandpas and grandmas. One lives far away and the other lives here. In the summer I live far away and during school I live here."

How did she like that? "It is great", she replied. "It is nice weather up there in the summer and nice here in the winter. I don't like snow."

The grandmother explained that 3 years ago the grandparents all got together and decided to raise her using this split year arrangement. Soon the lab results came back and she was discharged with medicine dispensed for strep throat. She was such a well-adjusted girl.

****

The story told by the mother of a 19-day-old baby had the staff worried. The baby was having periods of "not breathing after gagging and vomiting white curdled substance." An apnea (breathing) monitor was ordered from OB and applied in the ER.

While a few simple tests were being completed, the mother was advised not to feed the baby since milk may be the cause of the problem. A few minutes later she was found breastfeeding the baby. The nurse who observed this stated in a serious tone, "Put that thing away, here is a bottle of water if the baby is thirsty." Mother's reply was that the baby was crying and would stop if given breast milk.

During the admit report the mother's name brought an "Oh, no" reply from the nurse in OB. This mother had called every day since she went home after birth about problems with the baby. Some days it was 3 or 4 times. Just 36 hours ago the doctor ordered abdominal x-rays because of all the complaints. The tests concluded nothing was wrong except the baby was being overfed. Every time there was a whimper or cry or grunt there would be a bottle or breast shoved into the baby's mouth. At regular feedings, the mother would follow up the breastfeeding with another 4 ounces of formula. It was after these excess feeding sessions that gagging and vomiting of all the excess milk came back up. The lack of breathing was a result of gagging but only lasted a few seconds. In the mother's mind the lack of breathing must have seemed a lot longer.

The mother and baby were taken to the OB department for them to deal with education sessions for the mother. Good luck on that.

****

Her protruding lower lip was almost comical as a 5 year-old girl was brought in on a cot from the ambulance. She was really mad. She had a history of seizures for the past year and had a small seizure earlier at home. Her older sister knew what to do and put her on the floor in the middle of the room to let the seizure complete. When EMS arrived at the home, the youngster was in a sleepy state.

Walking beside the cot was her 13 year-old sister, who had been babysitting while the parents had gone to the grocery store. The ambulance crew contacted her parents in order to obtain permission to treat the girl. The time it took to get permission allowed the child to become fully awake. EMS tried to take her vital signs but she was combative and got mad, resulting in the protruding lower lip. They decided to just bring her in as she was, since she appeared stable.

Soon the parents arrived in the ER, resulting in a changed attitude and the lower lip went back to normal. From then on, she was the most sweet and loving little girl. Her parents described her mental condition as "slow development" with the capacity of a 2 year-old still in diapers.

After a blood test for her anti-seizure medicine was in normal range, they were advised to follow up with their doctor for medication adjustment.

A side note: The household consisted of 4 children, of which 3 have seizure disorders and 2 are "slow development". The parents have their hands full.

Most 2 year-old girls have soft and intriguing eyes but one evening brought a patient with eyes full of mischief and trouble. At home it was those eyes the mother saw when she came into the room and found her playing with a nasal decongestant spray bottle. She had been trying to fill mommy's contact lens container with the spray. When asked what she was doing she replied, "Getting a drink." Her face was wet and the bottle was empty, which were the two reasons why they were in the ER. Mother's concern was the harm the decongestant could do to a baby if swallowed.

The grin on this girl's face was saying, 'I caused all this excitement? This is fun.'

Since humans ingest the spray into the nose without worry the question of harm was not an issue. But could there be side effects in larger quantities since it was not known if, or how much, the girl had ingested? The Poison Control Center did state that in larger quantities it could cause drowsiness, lower blood pressure, and a slowing of the heart rate.

The ER's treatment order was careful observation of the small, active and mischievous little girl. She got into anything and everything for a full 2 hours. Her mother did the best she could to keep the girl out of trouble but the staff had to help most of the time. It was obvious the drowsiness, lower blood pressure, and slow heart rate would not be an issue. She was sent home with the assumption that she had not actually ingested any of the nasal spray or at least not enough of it to hurt her. It was a long observation, but the patient was well. That was the most important part.

The most dreaded moment in ER would be an adult coming through the door with a limp baby who had dusky blue skin color. Especially if it were a 15 day-old premature baby with a screaming, crying mother. All this was enough to make the staff go into action like at no other time. The body of this baby was so small he was carried to the trauma room in one hand while tiny puffs of air mouth-to-mouth breathing were performed. Luckily in this case the skin was still slightly warm and hopes were high. Oxygen was quickly applied.

Three minutes of high flow oxygen were pushed into the lungs with a bag squeezed by a respiratory therapist. The skin started to change to a pink color. The breathing pattern was retracted, meaning each occasional voluntary inhalation caused the stomach to cave inward. The IV could only be obtained by putting a special needle into the bone marrow through the lower leg bone, which was smaller than the chicken drumstick bones on which we had practiced. Such a tiny patient.

After lab blood was drawn, the fluids were infused rapidly. It did not take much fluid since it was calculated by weight and he only weighed a few pounds. This was followed with a chest x-ray. By that time the tiny patient was fully pink, alert with open eyes and seemed to be looking at all of us. Cheers shattered the tension.

The chest x-ray revealed pneumonia in the right lung. That is not good in such a tiny baby with undeveloped lungs. The ambulance was called and the pediatric specialist contacted at an advanced hospital. All the transfer arrangements were made to get this patient to the PICU (pediatric intensive care unit).

A follow up call the next day stated the baby was touch and go all that night. Every time they tried to suction the 'junk' out of the lungs the skin would turn blue again. By morning it started to do some good without the skin color change. It was a good guess that within a week or so this tiny little child should be going home.

Just think about it – this baby was born 4 weeks before full gestation of 40 weeks and was now only 2 weeks old. That meant the patient who we saved should not even have been born for 2 more weeks.

****

A 16 month-old boy was brought in by his mother with a story about the child had started to fall off the couch and the mother grabbed his arm to prevent the fall. Since then the baby would periodically cry but continually refused to move his arm. Mother was extremely distressed thinking she had done something terrible.
After some simple tests like trying to move the arm or getting the child to move the arm it was determined it must be "nursemaid elbow'.

The little tyke was such a trooper, really trying not to cry, but would give a serious look to whoever came close to that arm. Sort of a 'do not touch my arm' look. He would cry a little then look into mom's eyes for help then look back at the intruder. It became a game – slightly extend a hand toward the arm and wait for the snap of the boy's head with that glaring look. This game of "reach and glare" did not help the situation when the doctor came into the room to do the "deed".

The normal procedure was to hold the forearm in one hand and wrap the other hand around the elbow. This caused the boy to really start glaring and crying and looking at mother. With a trained, quick twist it was all over. The boy stopped crying since he was able to move his arm without difficulty or pain.

A confirming x-ray was taken before discharge and all were happy. Even then, no one was allowed to touch that arm due to that controlling glare.

$$************************$$

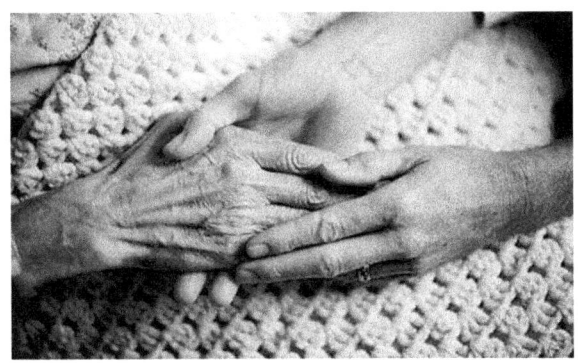

ELDERLY

Communication with a patient is important for good medical care in the ER. . This means providing full and accurate information on history, medications, recent happenings, current location of pain, and its' type and intensity. These are compromised with the care of elder patients. Other factors like heart rate and breathing are likely to be different from the norm in the older population.

Elderly patients brought into the ER present more challenges then most other ages. Dementia, Alzheimer's, physical disabilities, hearing difficulties, memory problems, poor eyesight and many more variables can make assessing and treating an elderly patient difficult. Many times they will deny pain no matter how many times they are asked about it. The following patients are probably the most profound of these types of cases.

****

A lady in her 80s was normally in good health and never had been in the ER before. Her sister stated she was not feeling well and her blood pressure was higher then normal on their home monitor. This person looked her age, appearing outwardly calm, but soon revealed that inside she was under a lot of stress.

The prim, proper lady seemed to carry herself well even though some spine problem made her walk bent forward. The limp had occurred after she tripped over a rug a few days ago, and must have sprained her knee, but it had not been checked out. She wore a floor-length dress with a jacket appearing fresh and well- ironed, as so many older people continue their grooming exactly as they have done all their lives.

She said she lived alone and two days ago her cat of 17 years had died. Also her best friend next door had died the week before. They had visited each other every day and now she had nobody, not even her cat.

Her blood pressure was confirmed as being critically high, but the diagnosis of anxiety was the source. A medication for stress and anxiety was given with good results. Her sister stated she would stay with her for a few more days. The patient replied, "You had better learn to 'meow' to make me feel better."

****

"There is some pain in my knee", was the only complaint of something being wrong. It came from a 79 year-old lady who had used her walker on a wood floor in stocking feet. She slipped, landing on her knee. Her son, with whom she lived, stated she tried to say nothing was wrong and had helped her into bed following the fall. He insisted she get checked out at the hospital.

Even in the ER she said softly that she was fine and wanted to go home. When she was allowed to sit on the edge of the bed and attempted to get up, she could not bear weight on the injured leg.

She had a guilty look and went on to say in a weak voice that she had fallen other times in the past week because "My legs buckled under". "Did they buckle because there was pain?" The answer was a faint and subdued, "Yes". The doctor assessed the knee by holding it up and moving it around. She told the truth at that point by loudly proclaiming, "DOC, YOU'RE KILLING ME!" It was hard to believe this meek lady could yell that loud.

The doctor had the son hold his hand on top of the kneecap, while moving the lower leg a little. The son became pale and almost passed out. He heard and felt the grinding of bone on bone called "crepitus". The patient told the doctor in no uncertain terms not to do that again. She was admitted for a fractured kneecap.

****

She was a sweet, soft-spoken 93 year-old lady with a pale

face, full of wrinkles on top of wrinkles, and a full head of silky smooth white hair. Her son, who was also soft-spoken, told the story of finding her lying on the floor of her kitchen. He guessed she had been there for at least 4 hours since she lived alone. He had asked her why she was on the floor. The reply was, "Cause I wanted to".

Typical of the elderly, she first refused to go get checked out by either her doctor or the hospital. Instead, she was put into her bed, but could not get the strength to get up except to use the bedside commode with help from her son. The strength, what little she did have, did not return to normal by the next day resulting in her arrival to the ER by ambulance.

All tests completed indicated nothing out of the norm except her potassium level was rather low. The doctor told her she had to be admitted for observation and a tune up. She replied, "Why would you want to do a "tune up"?

His reply echoed her previous phrase, "Cause I wanted to".

****

The paperwork had not arrived with an 85 year-old nursing home patient who had fallen out of bed complaining of left hip pain. The ambulance report included that the left leg was shorter and rotated inward, signs of either a dislocated hip or a hip fracture. X-rays were taken, indicating both left and right artificial hips were in their correct places with no fracture. The diagnosis was bruising of the hip.

The question remained as to why the left leg was shorter and rotated inward. Lots of questions were asked of the patient until she "remembered" she had scoliosis, a curvature of the lower spine. Sure enough, a closer inspection of her spine revealed a rather pronounced curvature making the entire pelvis tilt, resulting in a higher hip on the left. When asked why she did not tell of her back problem when asked so many questions about her shortened leg she replied, "I just forgot and besides, you don't have to know EVERYTHING about me".

She was admitted for a work-up to find a possible reason for falling out of bed, and to check on a long list of other ailments that were part of the long awaited paperwork that later arrived from the nursing home. Sure enough those papers listed hip replacement history.

****

A 60 year-old man was walking across the farmyard in the dark with a briefcase. A vintage pump handle "grabbed my knee and I fell to the ground." Because of the briefcase he was not able to catch his fall with his hand or arm, resulting in a face first contact with grass and dirt.

He broke his nose, causing a lot of blood splatter across his face and head. It looked worse then it really was. During the stitches on his nose he was jokingly telling stories about more recent "dumb" accidents and falls.

This became a concern resulting in a cat scan of his brain. The diagnosis was a tumor in his brain causing loss of coordination. As in so many ER cases the final diagnosis was not known, as to it being malignant or benign. Maybe that pump handle will not "trip" him again.

****

She weighed only 90 pounds with sunken cheeks and eye sockets. The nursing home sent this compliant frail lady in by ambulance due to injuries from a fall 4 hours earlier. The paperwork listed pain in the left shoulder and left hip. Medical history was diabetes, dementia, and lung cancer. They had picked her up from the floor and placed her in the bed. Due to advanced dementia she was unable to communicate her pains. When they moved her left arm she would cry. They decided it must be her shoulder and called for an ambulance.

In ER the hip had an obvious bruise under that transparent paper-thin skin, but the x-ray did not show any bone damage. It was the shoulder pain that could not be confirmed until the ER assessment indicated the pain was actually in the wrist. They must have held onto the wrist to facilitate the movement of the whole arm, resulting in a cry of pain. X-rays confirmed they had been holding a broken wrist and each movement of the arm caused a lot of pain. The lab test results came back showing a red blood cell count low enough to warrant two units of blood. They also found she was incontinent, her bowels resulting in black stool, indicating the presence of possible internal bleeding.

46

The whole time spent in ER this little lady stared fixedly into the eyes of any staff member working near her, almost like a plea for help. It was a helpless feeling since her advanced dementia allowed only cries and grunts for communication. It seemed she was trying to talk with her eyes. Most agreed she was doing just that, but it was difficult to understand.

Her wrist was put into a cast and then she was admitted for further treatments, including the needed blood transfusions and to find out where her internal bleeding may be. No wonder she was frail.

****

"One side of my face is numb". At least that was what it seemed to the 67 year-old gentleman who was "forced" to come to the ER by his family. This evening he had mentioned the occasional numbness to his daughter for the first time adding it had happened a couple of other times since his bypass heart surgery a few months ago. He had not told his extremely upset wife "making it necessary" for them to have it checked out "right in the middle of our vacation". He was at a loss to object since the two women were making the decisions.

The whole family came into the ER with great concerns for grandpa's emergency. His skin was a reddish color accented by multiple deep wrinkles common for a man with lots of outdoor adventures. He said he had gained "some" weight since the heart surgery, due to less activity and increased eating. He also confessed that he was not participating in the cardiac rehabilitation program at home. When asked about stress and anxiety he denied anything "really" bothered him.

His daughter surmised the reddish tint of his skin might be from "altitude sickness" in these Ozark Mountains. They were from Alabama with an altitude of 600 feet and she was shocked that she was sitting at only 800 feet above sea level. The patient had a distinctive big grin while enjoying the embarrassment shown by his daughter.

Tests were all negative, except his blood pressure was critically high. An anti-anxiety medication corrected that. At the

same time his reddish skin color and numbness was resolved.

Upon discharge he did admit he worried a lot about his heart condition since the bypass surgery, and had not slept well since then. He was advised to go to cardiac rehab back home and not to travel to "high altitude" places any more. That special grin reappeared.

****

About her 72 year-old husband's breathing, the wife said, "Breathing is supposed to be a quiet thing!" His inhalation had the very distinct sucking sound of a straw being used to get the last drop off the bottom of the glass. Expiration was a loud groan or moan like that heard mostly in a haunted house. She said, "I can't take it any longer. It's been going on for three days."

Her husband was barrel-chested from years of chronic obstructive pulmonary disease (COPD) and had a reddish colored skin, especially across the forehead. Temperature was 103 to accompany his body shaking like a leaf in a storm. He had been to the VA clinic for difficulty breathing about 10 days ago and was told he had "viral bronchitis". Proper medications were taken for the next 7 days that controlled his breathing problems. When the medications were completed, previous problems came back worse then before. His wife kept insisting he should go to the hospital but he was stubborn like most elderly men and women.

He was diagnosed with bilateral pneumonia (both lungs) and admitted to the hospital. On hearing the diagnosis, the wife gave a loud sigh of relief and turned to the patient and told him he should have listened to her. The doctor reminded her of her own words, "Breathing is supposed to be quiet". She gave the doctor a side-glance he recognized as not being appreciated.

A few days later the patient was observed being discharged and breathing quietly, but his wife was still making lots of noise telling him to listen to her. She obviously did not take her own advice that "breathing should be quiet."

****

Stubborn, independent, and arrogant pretty well described the 89-year-old woman brought into the ER by her neighbor of 20 years. Her first terse statement was, "She made me come in tonight. Gracie knows it is the best night for my TV programs and she wouldn't let me stay home. Get me out of here, fast. I am already missing one of those shows."

"Gracie" explained that the patient had been having episodes of chest pain for the past 3 days and refused any medical help, saying it was indigestion. Tonight it was more severe and she became scared for her friend's life. After many minutes of insisting she go to the ER, the stubborn gal finally gave in "just to get it checked and that is all!"

The first thing required was an IV and blood draw. Her derisive comment was "OK, you got it. I'm going home, and after you check it out call me if you need me to come back." When told she had to wait for the results her voice rose an octave, saying, "What do you mean I have to wait here - that is time wasted!" She finally consented to wait after many minutes of convincing, but "you only have a half hour". Of course it was longer than that, and more salesmanship was needed to make her stay.

The lab results indicated an elevated enzyme count that told us she had probably had a series of small heart attacks over the past few days. This meant she had to be admitted. She said it was impossible to do that tonight because, "I have some things to get done first, and besides it doesn't hurt anymore".

After she was informed there would be a TV of her own in her hospital room, she agreed to stay if it was done fast. "I had better not miss my other TV show." She was quickly admitted to the cardiac unit for more testing and monitoring. She demanded that she watch the show before the nurses did their check in process. Soon she said in disgust, "It is a rerun. So go ahead and do your thing."

Later a brief visit from the ER nurse was made for the purpose of finding out how she was doing, and to apologize for not telling her sooner about TVs in the hospital. She quickly quipped, "Yaw' l should learn how to treat old people," followed by a wink. She was quite an independent woman.

****

About 2AM the ambulance brought in a 70 year-old lady from a bus tour group found lying on the motel room floor. She had a temperature of 102.7 and could not even remember what State she resided in, or where and why she was here. No medical history or medication lists were available since the tour leader did not come in with her. All she could speak was "jibberish" talk at a fast pace not understood by anyone.

Medication for fever was given and a whole battery of tests, including a urine sample, was completed. Her temperature slowly reduced to 99.8. She gradually became lucid and very talkative. It was as if she remembered every question she was asked earlier and now wanted to answer them in one sentence with one breath. On and on she chatted, filling in all the details plus details about the details. She had no memory of the past 6 hours since she had gone to bed. She did complain of groin pain and was given some medication to combat that.

The urine lab results did confirm suspicions of a urinary tract infection and a shot of antibiotic was given, with a prescription for more. She was discharged as she suddenly remembered "one more thing" that we might "need to know" about her. No thanks, her entire life and more had been well documented!

****

A southern gal was admitted to the ER via an ambulance transfer from the local parking lot of a motel where the tour group was staying. She was 76 years old with a deep-southern drawl most people would die to have. "This shoulder hurts "soooooooo" bad I could "dai." The accent was so melodious and sweet the temptation was to ask the question again and again, to just hear that sweet drawl in true southern style.

The injury resulted when this blessed elderly belle missed the last step coming down a stairway and landed on her right shoulder. It was not only dislocated but the head of the upper arm bone was cracked across the middle. It was a severe injury that would have caused pain of the highest degree in most all cases. This lady should have been screaming and hollering for pain meds from the very beginning. Instead morphine was given in the ER without a request from her and her only comment was, "You're so sweet to help little ol' me with my pain. It is a little better."

The wording of that statement was a good hint she did need some more pain medicine, and she got it. Of course, that made the southern drawl peek through the slurred sentences, not making much sense. Valium was added when the dislocation of the shoulder was

---

going to be put back in place. This precious lady kept right on talking about "sweet", "kind" and a lot of words not having any meaning whatsoever, with an ever sustained dreamy drawl. It was mesmerizing.

After the bone was in the correct place, the distinct accent became more understandable over the next two hours. Her words of appreciation got more understandable as the drugs wore off, indicating she was ready to be discharged. Her tour bus was leaving in just a few hours for home in Texas. It was going to be a rough ride home even with the powerful pain pills she was given. One thing for sure, she would be complimenting the bus driver for taking all those "huge" bumps in the road with such great expertise.

****

A spry elderly 81 year-old lady was in a parking lot returning her shopping cart to the storage area when she tripped. The cart landed on top of her, but she said she was not hurt. Bystanders would not let her get up and called 911. The ambulance obligingly had to strap her on a backboard with c-collar on her neck, taping her head to the board so it could not move.

In the ER she was rather loud and insistent that these "dumb" straps be removed "immediately because nothing is wrong with me". The doctor quickly came into the room, and at one point his groin came close to her restrained hand. She grabbed the front of his scrub pants rather firmly saying, "Do you hear me now?" He released all straps and tape but left the c-collar in place on her neck. He promised he would take it off immediately if the radiologist said the cervical spine was not injured. Half an hour later he kept his promise.

This lady did show some age in spite of the make-up covering most of her age spots and wrinkles. One thing for sure, nothing could take away the twinkle in her eyes. Her age was questioned, but the daughter who had arrived and now sat nearby confirmed it was correct. A knowing grin came on the patient's face along with a bigger twinkle of the eyes.

The doctor ordered a set of "orthostatic readings" to be done. While in the standing position the technician told this slender lady to be sure to tell him if she was dizzy so he could catch her to keep her from falling. She denied any dizziness, but immediately placed the back of her hand on her forehead in a distinct theatrical style and slowly fell into the arms of the tech. Her daughter stated how embarrassed she was that her mother would do such a thing. With a quick wink, she threw her head back with the long hair trailing, and said, "At my age I have to take advantage of every opportunity." The daughter threw up her hands in disbelief.

She was discharged and seemed to be skipping along out the door. What a woman!

****

A 70 year-old woman with a long list of illnesses on her records, including dementia, was transferred from a local nursing home with a report of fever and decreased responsiveness, a common pair. It was amazing that no fever medication was given to the patient at the nursing home. They called her doctor and he ordered the transfer. He probably assumed they would do the proper medication from protocol.

Her temperature was 102.9 degrees on arrival to the ER and immediately she was given medication without an ER doctor's order per protocol. Her blood was sent to the lab about the time she said she needed to go to the bathroom "really bad". A small amount was obtained for a lab sample after the bedpan was taken away. With a smile she said, " I wet the bed, is that OK?" The true dementia patient would just do it and smile.

The family stayed in the waiting room most of the time during the lab, cat scans, and other procedures. During this time her temp came down to 100 degrees and she would ask questions with a smile. "Can you remove this cuff on my arm?" No. "Can you be bribed?" Dementia patients would just grab and pull the blood pressure cuff. Also demands for service like; "Lower my head!" "Raise my head!" "Cover my feet!" "Get me a drink!" They were simple and needed requests, but she would do it with more smiles. (Dementia?)

She was admitted with 'sepsis of the urinary tract'. On the way upstairs she became insistent she get a foley catheter, "So I will not wet the bed, plus I need 2 sleeping pills". These demands continued in front of the floor nurses and within earshot of her family in the hallway. The nurse that transferred her to the room asked, "You're going to be a pain in the neck for these nurses, aren't you? " She got a big grin and said, "Yep." The nurse kept playing her along, "What do you want next? - Wine?" Her reply, "Nope, a beer." There was a gasp from the hallway and then a snicker followed by laughter. She continued, "Make that 2 beers."

Dementia? Maybe so, and she was just having one of those "good days!"

****

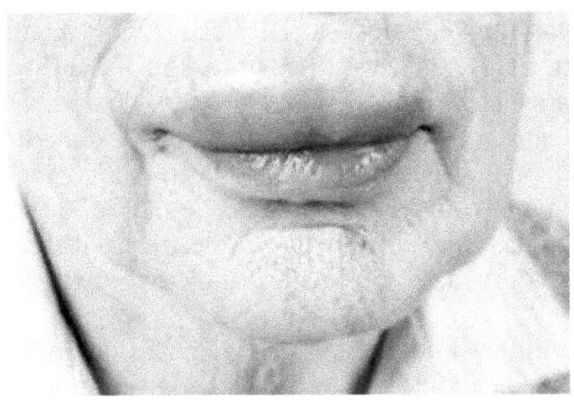

ALLERGIC REACTION

Allergic reactions can be a skin rash and/or swelling of hands, feet, face, tongue, and/or most any other part of the body. There is no cure for these reactions but the undesirable symptoms such as itch or swelling can be reduced. This allows for a more comfortable way for the body to fight off the foreign agent that the patient ate, inhaled, or got on the skin. It normally takes 3 to 4 days for the body to metabolize, neutralize, and excrete the "antigen". In the meantime, the medications prescribed are mainly antihistamines to lessen the itch, rash and swelling. It is common that the cause is never known.

If the tongue or lips are swollen there may be a need to keep checking for complications that could cause death due to asphyxiation by a swollen throat not able to be seen. An itchy rash on the skin causing a non-life- threatening condition is the most common type of allergic reaction seen in the ER. All that is usually needed is the standard treatment and then, discharge.

Treatments in most cases are these. First, a small shot of epinephrine; second, either a couple of antihistamine pills by mouth or the equivalent by IV; and third, sometimes a shot of an immune steroid. In the cases below these treatments were followed.

****

A 64 year-old lady came in with her upper lip swollen. It was so huge it almost hid the nostrils from view. Her demeanor was one of embarrassment about her looks. She was an attractive woman with expertly applied makeup and carried herself with matronly posture and confidence. 'Ugly' was the word she used to describe her current appearance.

A clue for a cause in this case was a new lipstick she had started to use a couple of days ago. She had been told a reaction would happen within a few hours after the first time used. It was explained different products and different people react differently. She accepted it was probably the lipstick and to be safe she threw it in the trash.

She was treated, got a lot better, observed, and let go with orders to continue the medication for 4 to 5 days. Her parting comment was that she would return when she looked normal to show us she really was not "ugly."

****

A 68 year-old man came in with his tongue swollen to the point that it would no longer fit in his mouth. He could breath through his nose but a close watch still had to be done every few minutes for possible airway blockage in the throat. If he opened his mouth as wide as possible he could take an oral breath - but it was a struggle. This plump balding man was rather quiet. Panic was common in cases where breathing was difficult, but this patient didn't panic and compliments were continually given to keep him that calm.

It is called "angioedema" - or a swelling reaction to 'something' that he came in contact with, or ate. Treatment helped to reduce the tongue size in about 3 hours. After another hour of observation he was released with more meds to be taken for at least 4 to 5 days. His wife was apprehensive about leaving, but the patient patted her on the shoulder for reassurance as they went out the door.

****

A 30 year old came running into the ER with her entire face looking like a balloon. Her eyes were just slits, her nose was only a knob, and her mouth was puckered up as if to give kisses. Her skin was like an advanced case of measles due to a rash. She was treated and then admitted, for possible further complications of swelling to the airway. The follow up the next day indicated most all the swelling was gone, and a beautiful face appeared. She was a dancer in a music show using a lot of makeup for the stage show. Could be a clue to the cause.

****

A 70 year-old came walking in with angioedema of the tongue. He awoke about 2AM with his tongue swollen to the point of barely protruding outside the mouth. His lips were ruby red and he complained they itched. He was not having any breathing difficulty but could not figure out what may have caused it. The patient was very anxious but finally relaxed when he was told a lot of these kinds of allergic reactions were seen over the course of the year and treatment had never failed to reverse the process.

His repeated question was about the cause. He would not accept the answer that it could not be determined and no test would be done to try to determine the cause. Only a dermatologist with lots of testing on the skin could make the 'best guess' as to the cause of an allergic reaction. He finally accepted this explanation about the same time his swelling disappeared and the red lips became normal. He said they still had an itch.

He was sent home with instructions to take the medicine every 6 hours for 4 to 5 days. Also, he was warned the pills would make him sleepy so naptime would be common. He was guardedly happy but his wife was joyous.

****

A 28 year old was brought in having severe abdominal pains with lots of nausea and vomiting plus a blotchy reddish color over most of his body. He was writhing and moaning, his body curled up so much there was no way to get a good history. An IV was started to give a nausea and pain med. It did not help. An anxiety medicine was given and that seemed to settle him down.

The high-pitched whining cry earlier was replaced with a deep calm voice. He was now able to tell us his actions for most of the day including all foods eaten. He ate a coconut donut (something new to him) and about an hour later he started getting hot flashes and a burning feeling, then the nausea and vomiting started.

The doctor gave a big, "Ah Ha! An allergic reaction to coconut!" A medicine via an IV was given, and soon his nausea lessened and the pain subsided. It had been a full four hours since he arrived and another two hour being treated in the ER. The possible return of his previous symptoms was a concern. Besides the robust looking man was totally wiped out and sleeping like a helpless baby. He was admitted for observation.

****

A middle aged, pleasantly plump lady came in with nausea, vomiting and diarrhea saying it was probably from some restaurant food she had eaten earlier. The usual questions regarding allergies to any medications got a negative response. An IV was started to give an anti-nausea medicine. The IV was also used to pump a lot of fluids in to replace the loss from the vomiting and diarrhea.

In this case, she did not know it but she was extremely allergic to the anti-nausea medicine given. She started to curl her hands and arms tight, shake almost like a seizure with eyes rolling back, mouth spewing foam, and all kinds of gyrations. This was an emergency because she could vomit again and breathe in at the same time, causing emesis in the lungs. Normally a dose an anti-histamine IV will start the cure but not with this lady. She was strong and restless with jerky spasms and anxiety. She could not talk but probably could hear.

Another 2 drugs were given with some effect. She stopped the grand movements and just jerked her body every once in a while. After being admitted to intensive care it was reported that she fell asleep. A case of the initial "cure" was worse then the original sickness. Her medical records would now record she was allergic to at least one medication."

****

A 30 year-old man got a new job. His first few hours went fine but he then started to feel tightness in his throat. This continued for a while and then he had a feeling of "my lungs are collapsing" and it was getting harder to breathe, which added to the anxiety.

Being in no real distress at the moment he arrived in the ER and a few background questions were asked of which one was, "Are you allergic to anything?" His reply was, "Yes, shellfish".

He was treated for an allergic reaction, which did improve

his condition, and he relaxed. He was asked, "Oh, by the way, where is this new job?" His reply was, "Red Lobster". What was he thinking?

****

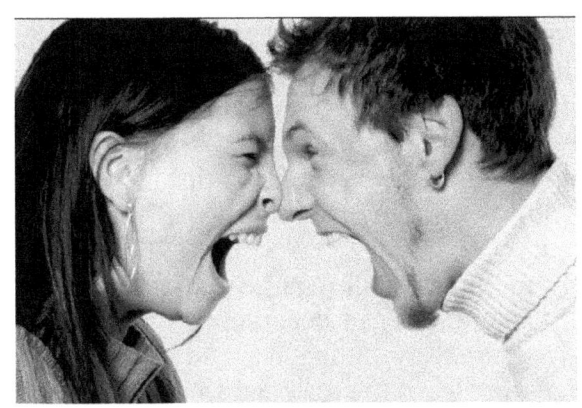

ABUSE

Alcohol was the main catalyst for most abuse cases that came to the ER. It seemed improbable that one or two persons would have been able to inflict such mean and violent acts on one another without it's influence. Most victims were women, but occasionally it was the reverse. The patients went from the very beautiful looking to the polar opposite. They were tall, short, skinny, fat, and all skin colors. An observation – most of the physical abusers were husky and had more than one tattoo.

****

The ambulance arrived with a 40-ish gal sporting a short haircut, no shoes, glasses, or watch but her clothes intact and she was wearing a wedding ring. She had been found stumbling along the major highway with an abrasion on one arm and her nose was swollen with dried blood visible inside both nostrils. There were no scalp injuries, easily noted due to the short hair. She was missing most of her teeth on the left side and later she said her denture was at home. A close look at the left cheek inside and out indicated swelling to twice the normal thickness.

During the physical exam she cried and sobbed a story that she was in a pickup truck with her husband and adult son on either side of her. An argument between all three about drunk driving ended with her decision to walk home even though she herself had been drinking. "I struck my cheek and nose on the dash getting up and over my son and out of the truck." It was at this point the infamous phrase was heard loud and clear between sobs, "It was all my fault." She denied either husband or son did anything to her.

Blood tests and urine tests came back while she was in radiology having a cat scan and x-rays. Her blood alcohol was 3 times the legal limit to drive. The urine drug screen indicated marijuana. The patient came back to the ER room more composed and less sobbing.

Shortly the police took charge and asked all the questions. She eventually admitted it had been her son who had kicked her in the cheek.. He started by hitting her with his fist so the husband pulled onto the shoulder of the road and stopped to let her get out per her request. Hitting continued as she tried to get out, striking her head on the dash and then falling out onto the ground. After more screaming back and forth for a few minutes she tried to get back into the truck. It was then the son kicked her in the left cheek, resulting in her fall and scraping her arm on the pavement. Both husband and son were hollering that she could walk home as they sped off down the highway.

The cat scan results revealed multiple fractures of most of the left facial bones, upper jaw, eye sockets, sinus bones and nose. In short the injuries were extensive and would require surgery.

She said she was going to press charges and move out but it almost never seems to happen. She was admitted to the intensive care unit with the sheriff's deputies leaving to make the arrest of her husband and son. She never let go with blaming herself for what happened.

****

It was just above freezing outside at 3:30AM when the ambulance radio report stated they were in route to the ER with a 40 year-old female found walking and stumbling along the county road barefoot without a coat, wearing only blue jeans and tee shirt. She was alert but could not remember anything except it was still light outside when she started to feel cold. There was dried blood on her clothes and face but no active bleeding at the time. The conclusion was that she probably was a victim of assault, but she could only say, "I am cold". The report also included vital signs close to normal, except a temperature of 93.1 degrees.

On arrival she was stripped of all clothing and placed under a special blanket with warm air blowing thru tiny holes onto her skin. She was shaking like a leaf on a cottonwood tree during a storm. Her arms and hands were so cold an IV could not be started. After 20 minutes of warm air her temp was 95.8 degrees and an IV was obtained. Warm saline fluid was pumped rapidly into her veins to increase the core temperature and mental orientation.

This rather pretty blond haired lady started to remember there had been an argument and altercation at her daughter and son–in–law's home when she was told to get out. She went home depressed and took some sleeping pills with a whole bottle of liquid Nyquil. How many pills – her best recollection it was an "almost new bottle of 24". This was a drug overdose case, and appropriate treatment was started with an antidote called MucoMist.

There were bruises starting to form on the underside of both forearms indicating she held them in front of her face to protect from blows being struck. Therefore, assault was added to the picture. When asked if she was married she said, "Yes, for 20 terrible years".

This lady was admitted to intensive care for more MucoMist treatments to prevent a painful, horrible death from liver failure due to acetaminophen overdose, plus counseling, and hopefully a new life. She became quiet and expressed a
lot of gratefulness to the ER staff for being so compassionate to her.

Was the assault from her husband or daughter? As in
so many ER cases, the end of the story was never known.

****

A 52 year-old man was brought in by ambulance from an assault. He had a lot of bruises and sore spots and a few scrapes - but x-rays indicated there were no broken bones. He reported that his daughter and her boyfriend had beaten him, even kicking him while on the ground.

He briefly got some sympathy even though his blood alcohol was 0.22, which might have been his normal level all the time since he admitted he was an alcoholic. When getting ready to discharge him, the police showed up saying they would like to talk to him. He was in violation of his parole. He had assaulted his wife that morning. His daughter had been getting even for his treatment of her mother.

****

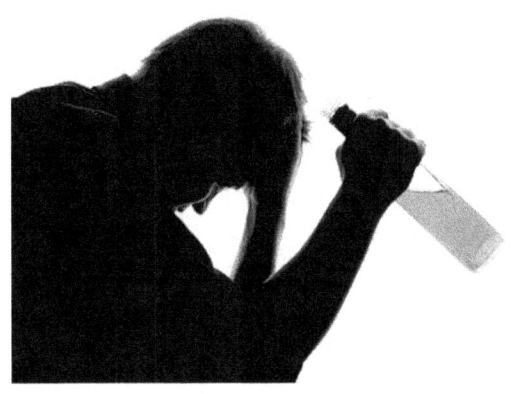

DRUNKS

Men and women of every social strata, rich and poor, homeless and homeowners, legal or illegal, will from time to time drink to excess. Some of the time there are side effects and consequences directly or indirectly related to the over indulgence of alcohol. In some of the cases, the emergency room is called upon to resolve the situation, or at least provide some semblance of normalcy. Sometimes drunken patients are quiet, but others can be combative protesting loudly about just being at a place they think is not necessary.

The medical staff has to be flexible in the attitude category. Sometimes a protesting patient needs an angry and demanding doctor to bring control. Others may need a soft sympathetic voice. If one does not work, we try the other one. With each drunk that arrives either by ambulance or private car, it is at times frustrating, since the complications are not as clear as, perhaps, a trauma patient with cuts and scrapes. A drunk can have serious injuries but may not know that fact since alcohol numbs the senses. ER must become those senses to determine the best treatment.

****

The police dispatcher heard on the scanner was having an ambulance dispatched to the jail for a combative and hyperventilating female. Soon, an officer arrived in the ER, ahead of the ambulance, to inform us that she was under arrest for drunken driving for the 4th time. The next bit of information came from the ambulance report, stating she was calm, non-combative with no complaints. What changed?

This information required a revision of the pre-plan to a new pre-plan. If she arrived with no complaints then we would have a "permit to treat" form ready for her to sign. It must be filled out listing a chief complaint. If she does not have one, then we would offer an AMA (against medical advice) form prior to discharge. All this, even before a temperature could be taken. Upon refusal, she would then be eligible to go right back to jail.

On arrival the obviously drunk middle-aged gal with messed up hair, smeared lipstick and runny eye makeup was calm. Before signing, she insisted on reading the one-page 'consent to treat' form containing all kinds of legal terms. After stumbling verbal attempts to 'read" it all, she could not remember what her "chief complaint" was that had brought her here. The whole process was humorous, but the laughs and giggles had to be suppressed to keep the patient's attention on the paper and not on being an entertainer. She finally "remembered" it was "chest pain."

When it came time to get her signature at the bottom of the form, she looked around and said she wanted to pick out the person who would do the examination. A young male technician was pointed out to be her "caregiver." She would not permit anyone else except the doctor. It was decided to go along with her to keep the peace.

With an RN close by, the technician completed the total of all assessments as far as she was concerned. Every time he came close, she would start making overt suggestions about the two of them, which he handled quite well. An example was when she was to have an EKG for her heart and refused, his reply was, "Prove to me you have a heart, and we will talk."

It was not long until the patient was napping, with deep snoring. All tests came back negative during this time and she was released to go back to jail. She was asked if she wanted to say goodbye to her "love-of-my-life nurse." She did not remember anyone like that. The technician gave a big sigh of relief.

****

Getting drunk usually led to added complications as an older man found out, according to the story he told the EMTs. The moonless night made the night so dark it had been hard to see anything. He was drinking liquor straight from the bottle with others on the shoreline of a local lake when he passed out, only to awaken all alone. Thinking his drinking buddies were nearby he stumbled around looking for them but passed out, falling into the water. The outside temperature was near freezing and it was not known how much time passed before a passerby found him half reclined in waist deep water. Due to a lot of unknowns, the EMT's put this man on a backboard, c-collar and straps, to hold him on the board. Drunks dislike this safety precaution more than anyone else, and they usually fight it hard.

On arrival to the ER the task of stripping off all the wet clothing was facilitated with a pair of scissors. This increased the patient's bad attitude, which he would not even be able to remember in the morning. All he wanted was to get all the restraints off.

His loud screams of objection while submitting to a rectal thermometer made most of us think he was being slowly killed. The core temperature was 95.3 degrees so a hot air blanket was in place most of the time he was in the ER. X-rays of his neck were completed as quickly as possible. The excess energy spent fighting the collar and backboard must have helped burn off some of the alcohol in his system, since he was more coherent and calm after the restraints were removed.

When he became warmed and the hot air blanket was removed, he informed us he was from a town 50 miles away and had no one here to pick him up. He had gotten a ride to town during the day and apparently missed his ride home. A sandwich and coffee were provided and clothes were furnished to him from the emergency supply kept in the hospital, but he could not be discharged into freezing temperatures. He had no money to get a cab. Finally a person from his hometown was contacted, and agreed to come get him but not until noon, 6 hours later. The decision was made to let him stay in the waiting room, where he slid down into the chair and immediately fell asleep. He was still sleeping quietly in the waiting room at shift change.

****

The police escorted a handcuffed, mildly inebriated middle-aged man into the ER stating he was under arrest for public drunkenness. The story given was during the process of arresting him the patient "bumped" his face on the ground causing a 1/8" cut on the lower lip. It bled profusely, which made the man very mad while accusing the police of brutality and demanding stitches. Most every screaming sentence had 2 or more words of profanity directed at the police who were still shouting orders at him without success. Soft words by the ER staff did not work. His demands, rebukes, and accusations were easily heard in the far corners of the department.

When the doctor came into the room, the patient did quiet down a little but kept talking. The doctor told him stitches could not be put into a lip laceration while it was moving. If he could shut up for a few minutes the procedure could begin. If he could not keep still, a drug would be given to temporarily "paralyze" him in order to get it done. The patient went ballistic saying this hospital was trying to take over the world by paralyzing everyone.

He resumed a profound profanity marathon that mainly said no one in this evil hospital was going to touch him. This resulted in a refusal of all care. The laceration did not really need a stitch, so his leaving in handcuffs with the police escort to go to jail was not something of concern. With him gone, the quiet throughout the ER seemed almost eerie!

****

A 35 year old man found staggering along the highway a few miles out of town was nowhere near any residences. The deputy related that he determined the man was just drunk and put him under arrest for public drunkenness. The word "jail" must have awakened him from his drunken stupor and he immediately complained of chest pain. He arrived at the ER by ambulance, moaning and groaning, but at least was not loud and profane. He did not have any ID and was not able to speak except a slurred first name that had to be repeated numerous times before anyone could understand it.

When we started IV fluids, more identification information was attempted. Periods of passing out, slurred words, blank stares and other drunken actions were the norm. After many events of passing out, a sternal rub with knuckles on the breastbone woke him more then usual. He suddenly remembered a girl's name. Another 5 minutes of asking who she was to him determined it was his baby daughter. Finally a phone number was obtained, just before the next flop of the head to the pillow in an unresponsive state.

The phone was answered by his ex-significant other, the mother of his 3 year old daughter. She stated that neither she, nor her daughter would have anything to do with him. At least the patient's name, date of birth and last known address was obtained. He was then found in the computer system with added people to contact. He would have someone to care for him once he got sober enough to be discharged.

****

An 80 year-old lady was found slow to respond on the kitchen floor at home. The official diagnosis was "syncopal episode" – the fancy name for passing out. What happened before this event was the interesting story.

The lady liked to have a few beers each evening. In fact, the daughter with whom she lived would limit her to only 2 cans of beer because of the chances of her drinking too much. The rest of the 6-pack was hidden from her. Each evening this happy, feisty woman would go out to the porch, sit in her rocking chair, sip her 2 cans of beer, and unfailingly ask for another one she never got. .

This night, the family had to run a short errand about the time the evening ritual was to start. They helped her get settled into the rocking chair and left. Little did they know she had found the stash of beer and quickly finished off the rest of the 6-pack. She put the empty cans back in the hiding place before passing out.

Upon returning home, the family said she was face down on the kitchen floor moaning, trying to speak with mumbling words. Thinking stroke they called the ambulance. The smell of beer on her breath was normal for this time of day so no suspicions were formed as to what really happened.

In ER her blood alcohol level was 20% and all tests and scans for other possibilities were negative. She did gain some semblance of normal conversation and "confessed" to her deed. She had a big smile during this conversation, since she knew she had gotten one over on the family. "There will be a new, locked hiding place," was the promise by the daughter.

****

It was a quiet night at 1AM when a man ran into the triage area stating his daughter was in the car, not breathing. Two people made a dash with a wheelchair to the ambulance bay, following the father. Security was also in the bay and quickly transferred a dishrag-limp 21 year-old gal to the wheelchair and made for the nearest trauma room. The commotion and shouts for a doctor brought 2 nurses, 2 doctors, 2 ER techs and 1 respiratory tech into the room at the same time. One quick heave moved the gal to the cot with a thud. There was no reaction from her. Weak respirations were heard and the pulse oximeter indicated 95% saturation, adequate for adults.

The greatest worry was she might aspirate some vomit into her lungs while unconscious. She gagged violently on the first intubation attempt and moaned as if to complain. She had to be sedated for the tube to be inserted into her lungs, and a 'breathing machine' was attached. Other tubes were inserted into other places to make caring for her easier and avoid embarrassment later on. Two high flow IV's were started to dilute the reported alcohol she had consumed.

Her father said he had come back into her life after an absence of 4 years that very day. He took her and her fiancé out to dinner, where she had drank wine. She passed out in the car on her way home. He said she might be taking diet pills that reacted to the alcohol.

Her mother arrived and added more to the story. The father had left with another woman and never contacted them or sent any money during his four-year absence.

About an hour later all tests were completed, showing a .211 blood-alcohol, which is high for a young gal that usually never drinks. The sedative drugs were also wearing off about this time and she was able to communicate. Removal of all the tubes was clearly indicated soon, but the doctor did not want to take a chance of aspiration so he left them in place as she was admitted to the CCU.

Later the report from the unit said she had all the tubes removed and was trashing her father. Even though she was out of it due to the alcohol, she could hear what was said earlier. She heard the "lies" her father said about the diet pills. She did not take any kind of pills and weighed only 125 pounds. She told everyone she did not want to see her father again.

How drunk could a person get? The highest witnessed blood alcohol in a person still able to talk and even stumble around was one night in the ER. A 38 year-old man was found unresponsive on the doorstep of the alcohol rehab center. It was assumed it was fellow alcoholics who drove him there preferring to remain unknown.

He arrived at ER by ambulance, combative and not wanting anyone to even touch him. The words stumbled past his lips in a jumbled mess but the bad intentions were fairly clear. After some hot coffee and a bite of sandwich, he settled down to allow a blood draw. The result was a 0.556 blood alcohol. All books teach anyone over 0.40 is comatose unless a chronic alcoholic was involved, as was obvious for this patient.

For the next 6 hours, IV fluids were the order of the night. After 3 quarts the blood alcohol was 0.466, just .066 points from the requirement for admit to the rehab center. The patient was calm, agreeable, and rather funny at this point. He ate 3 sandwiches with milk, coffee, and water while expressing lots of gratitude. At first he did not want to go to the rehab center because that had been tried 5 times in the past. Later he was convinced it was the best thing to at least try again. He was discharged to the rehab center with a blood alcohol of 0.38, walking a straight line, with words uttered in a somewhat organized manner.

An ATV (all terrain vehicle) was this "hillbilly" resident's downfall, when he and a female friend went for a ride. He was dressed in bib overalls and a tank top shirt exposing lots of tattoos. It must have been his straw hat that defined his status. He was 45 years old and his riding partner was 27 years old. Her attire was short-shorts, halter top and barefoot. Both had been drinking from a clear bottle without a label.

A spin out followed, and both landed in a ditch and were taken by ambulance to the ER. The man was concerned about the condition of his female friend, since they were being put in separate rooms. After repeated requests about her status, a nurse went to the gal's room to make inquiry and to get permission to report back to the man. A deep voice, the kind that demands respect and makes some people quiver in their boots, replied to the request, "Who is asking?" If it is the (blank) driver of that ATV tell that (blank) it is none of his (blank) business!"

The hillbilly patient overheard, and from that point on asked nothing about the girl. Near the end of some stitches on his arms and face he did comment, "Oh, well - it was fun while it lasted - if that is the way it has to be - OK". Upon discharge, he asked for an exit that did not go past the room where she was located. He staggered and stumbled on his way to the waiting room, where a relative was ready to take him home.

****

The bar had just closed and all were in the parking lot making their way to cars. The unfortunate victim was a 160 pound 22 year-old "punk" who heard a rather large man insult his friend. He had been at the bar since 8PM and reportedly became more arrogant as the drinks were consumed.

A retaliatory assault on the "brute" was short and complete, leaving the young "punk" with a split lip from fists, and scrapes on the arms caused by sliding backward across the blacktop. Soon EMTS arrived, and it became a drunk's worst nightmare to be strapped to a backboard with c-collar and head restraints. Most all become violent when they cannot be freed from this bondage. This case was no exception.

On arrival to the ER he was combative and would not allow anyone to touch him until he could go to the bathroom. He had an almost constant chant of the need to "GO". X-rays and cat scans were needed to clear his spine and neck before the restraints could be removed. The solution was for him to urinate in his pants to get relief. That was impossible to perform spontaneously. In his altered state of mind, he could not understand the dangers of letting him turn and twist his head might put him into a wheelchair the rest of his life.

His altered reasoning was that being a quadriplegic might be a good thing. He would then be waited on hand and foot for all his needs. He was reminded of all the other problems like having to have a foley catheter, not able to have bowel movements easily, bed sores, drop foot and, of course, no sex. That did it. He promised not to resist any more and have all tests needed.

Shortly he was cleared of possible spinal damage and allowed to stand at the bedside to use a urinal. He filled the first one and made a good start on the second, an amount about twice the normal. He indeed needed to "go".

His blood alcohol was 0.32. His friend was in the ER, ready to take him home. After a few stitches in his lip and scrubbed abrasions on his arms, he left the ER with an arrogant stride that told all he knew he had lived through this one and would probably be back, after the next night at the bar and an insult to a friend.

****

It was early morning and a 30 year-old woman had been drinking with her "fiancée" at another couple's home. An argument resulted, and she took her 3 year-old son, got into her truck and drove off.

Shortly she crashed into a tree, with the steering wheel slamming into her lower abdomen. EMS reported she was lying on the ground outside the truck screaming about pain in the groin. Her son was in his car seat unhurt, not even crying.

She had a non-displaced pelvic fracture, internal bleeding and, of course, the burst bladder so common with drunk accident victims at this hour. Her tests indicated a blood alcohol of 0.21. Surgery was ordered immediately, and she would spend lots of time in recovery and rehabilitation plus probation and more.

Drinking for her that night was a quadruple loss. She lost her boyfriend, her truck, her driver's license and her son, as he became the custody of the State. In her altered mind condition the only comment to all this was, "Oh, well. Let's have another drink."

****

A middle-aged drunk came in not feeling good mainly because his blood alcohol was 0.33 on arrival. The next few hours of IV, food, and coffee helped to lower the level. Near shift end the attempts to get his wife to come pick him up were not successful. A taxi voucher was issued to pay for his trip home.

Conversations during the course of the night indicated there were some marital problems and she may not be home because of infidelities on her part. This situation was the reason he was drinking to excess that night. Lots of "good lucks" were given when he left for home, hoping she would be there on arrival.

The following night the same man arrived with the same alcohol problem. He explained upon arriving home that morning his duffel bag was sitting on the front porch with a note not to come back. He got back into the taxi and came back to town to drink his sorrows away. He was treated again and released to alcohol rehab to help get him back on track.

****

When a 33 year-old man was brought into the ER the ambulance report stated he smelled of alcohol and was combative. A "good" Samaritan found him lying on the ground and thought he was hurt so had called for help. He was resisting transportation saying he was just drunk. He refused to be treated and asked to sign out AMA.

The doctor in this case was known for her out of the ordinary ways of treating patients. Normally a doctor would assess the patient and agree he was probably drunk and nothing else was wrong, allowing the police to take him to jail for public drunkenness. Not this time, she reasoned he was too drunk to be able to make medical decisions for himself. She ordered a blood test, a urine test, and neck x-rays.

The whole staff was stunned when the patient refused to let them be done. She then ordered a 4-point restraint (both arms and legs) to facilitate her orders. It took 5 people, besides the restraints, to get the blood draw and the foley catheter for urine. In x-ray he moved at the wrong time (or in his mind the right time) resulting in a blur. He was sent back to his room without results. No drugs were found in the urine and his blood alcohol was 0.28.

To further "teach this patient a lesson" she said she noticed pavement dirt or scrapes along his left side. That meant a possible spleen injury requiring a cat scan. This meant drinking 12 ounces of a terrible tasting liquid 3 times in 2 hours. That was not going to happen as far as the patient was concerned. The doctor then ordered a tube be inserted into the nostril and extended to the stomach so the liquid could be poured in. If that did not work, she was planning on sedating him for intubation.

It was at this point the entire staff involved "went on strike" and refused to follow any of her orders. Also, it was known that she went off duty in about ½ hour and the new doctor would take over. She became irate that nurses would refuse to carry out a medical order. She did write a report to administration but the incident was not heard of again.

The new doctor assessed the patient, listened to the staff report, read the documentation by the other doctor, saw the lab reports, and decided the patient was tortured enough. It had been 5 hours of fighting the patient and the doctor but the right people won. He was the happiest drunk that ever left the ER in route to jail. Would he ever drink again? Probably so.

****

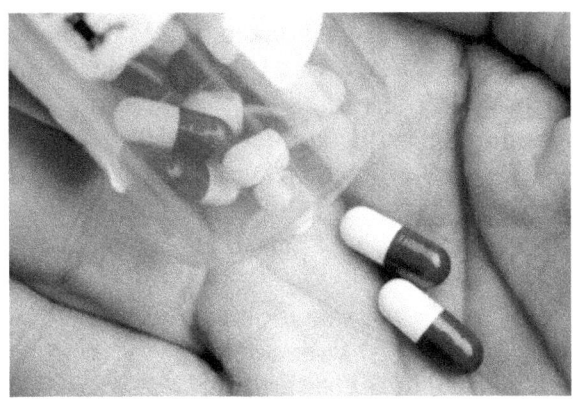

<u>DRUGS</u>

People from every walk of life get involved with drugs. ER involvement happens in two major ways. Sometimes people come in to get their "fix" by faking an injury and insisting on a strong pain killer for their "severe" injury. Most of the time, they ask for the specific drug by name, which gives away their motive. The second reason they come to the ER is for bad side effects caused by a drug, an overdose, or even the lack of a drug – like running out of a prescription. Here are a few incidents of the memorable people who came in seeking illegal drugs, or presented as a result of taking illegal drugs.

****

About midnight, a 24 year-old gal was picked up by ambulance in a known area for drug distribution and use. She was barely breathing when paramedics arrived. To assure an open airway, a nasal tube was inserted into her nostril without difficulty.

On arrival to the ER, her respirations were better and she had a strong pulse. Her arms and legs were limp with not a finger or toe twitching. She had the appearance of being dead but had acceptable vital signs. Painful stimuli such as a hard rub on the breastbone created no reaction. Her eyes were wide open, blankly staring at the ceiling. Her mouth was also wide open, and we heard an occasional snort or snore. The effect was sort of like being in Transylvania, waiting for a Dracula monster to sit up proclaiming life.

At the scene a witness had mentioned a sedative/pain-type

opiate drug, which may have been taken. Most people who take this drug say they feel lightheaded and dizzy while an overdose can cause hallucinations. A test did show the presence of that type of drug in her system, plus an alcohol level of 10 percent. A reversing medication was given through an IV, but her condition remained unchanged. The pupils remained fixed with that ghostly upward stare, not deviated even with a snap of the fingers or a clap of the hands.

This young gal with good-looking features did not appear to be a drug user. However, she remained on the bed in a very still manner, no matter which way her arms or legs were placed. Putting a tongue depressor in her mouth all the way to the throat would cause a gag reflex, and touching the eyelid would create a flutter. Every once in a while, we observed her eyelids blinking. When asked if she could blink her eyes once for yes and twice for no she blinked once to everyone's amazement.. The first question was a one blink answer, whether she had taken the drug, and we found out she had only taken one pill.

She was informed that if she needed anything to blink more then twice. Rapid blinking was the reply. An elimination process began. "Was it below the neck?" 2 blinks. "On the face?" 1 blink. "The mouth?" 2 blinks. "The nose?" 1 blink. "The tube in the nose?" 1 blink. "Want it out?" Many blinks. The airway tube was removed. "That better?" 1 blink. She answered other questions by rapidly blinking. One important concern she had was obtained after many elimination questions. "Am I going to die?" She was assured she was not going to die. Other meds were tried for a possible 'dystonic' reaction but they did nothing to improve her condition, at least during the time she was in the ER. She was admitted to intensive care.

The following noon, she was near normal with all functions working, and even took a walk down the hall. She did not remember anything from the ER except something about blinking her eyes a lot and that she was scared. It was not known, what caused her extreme reaction, but a drug mixed with alcohol was the most likely reason. When advised not to ever mix drugs and alcohol, she assured everyone it would never happen again. She was transferred for observation in a step-down room until the next day when she was discharged.

****

At 67, she was the matriarch of the family, commanding the respect of all her children and grandchildren in her simple, quiet way. During a vacation it was no different, as the family of 10 sat down at a table in the dinner theater. Just as the salad was served, this prim and proper lady suddenly started jerking and fell face first into the salad bowl. From there, it was a smooth slide off the table and chair onto the floor. So the story went, as told by her son.

On arrival to the ER by ambulance she varied between seizure and change in mental status. Normally the post seizure sleepiness does not last more then a few minutes, but this had lasted an hour. Besides, she had never had a seizure before. Since she was still "sleeping" with some audible moans and groans and unable to communicate, it was difficult to determine the possible cause. A blood test, heart test, brain test and more gave us no clues.

Gradually the "mental status" of this stately woman with perfectly combed white hair (smeared with salad dressing) started getting better. Her speech was garbled like a deep-sea diver, then slurred like a true drunk, and soon somewhat understandable. The blanks were starting to fill in. The only prescribed medication she took regularly was a nerve pill. However, she had forgotten them at home when she left 3 days ago on this vacation. She figured she could do without. Why not – here was a very capable woman, and to skip her medication should be nothing.

She learned that being the matriarch was tough but if nerve pills were needed it can be even tougher without them. She was diagnosed with a "benzodiazepine withdrawal" like an alcoholic having a withdrawal.

A small dose of that medication was given, plus a prescription to be filled. The family was glad they could continue their vacation, and now they were in charge as she temporarily lost her matriarchal status. Surely, she would be back in command shortly!

****

Some people came up with fantastic stories in order to get narcotic drugs in the ER. The stories were somewhat believable, but normally had enough inconsistencies to make it an unreliable source for their pain. Take the case of the 36 year-old male staying in town with his ex-in-laws. A clue right there, only a con man would be ableto stay with an ex-in-law.

The story of his injury was also suspect. He was riding "his" bike down a hill. Did he bring the bike into town with him? The truck ahead "slammed on his brakes causing the bike to collide with the rear end of the truck." The patient stated he flew into the top edge of the tailgate, hitting his ribs, then fell to the ground striking his right knee on the pavement. Of course the truck "sped off" without checking on the condition of the rider. This con man, now called a patient, was claiming severe pain in the ribs and right knee.

The story was not believable to the cops, the doc, or anyone who heard it. As a classic drug seeker in true form he kept asking for specifically named narcotic drugs. X-rays cleared all ribs and right knee from any specific disabling injury. Therefore he was offered Tylenol or Advil. He did scream and holler, threatening to sue and making other threats, but ended up leaving in a "huff". We all noticed he was not limping on exit.

****

How much of a drug would it take to cause death? This was the question a 16 year-old female had, after she had taken eight narcotic tablets with some vodka. She was at a party and decided to find out what it felt like to get a "drug addict high". Having no idea how many pills an addict would take, she chose whatever she had in her hand. Later, a friend told her she must be crazy because he "knew for a fact" that ten of those would kill you, and with booze it would take less. Panic set in, and after putting her fingers down her throat and vomiting only phlegm, she laid down on a couch and waited to die. She took a nap and awoke shocked to find out she was still there.

Still anxious to find out how long it would take before she died she was brought to the ER. She was informed immediately that the chances of dying were next to zero. The only possible thing to worry about was the acetaminophen contained in the medicine. It can damage the liver in high doses but, if lucky, not in the quantity taken by a healthy person such as herself. Her father was contacted and he gave permission to do whatever was needed to help her, not only physically but also mentally, to encourage her to stop her bad drug habits.

After the doctor did his normal assessment, he leaned back

against the counter in his patented posture for a serious lecture. First, she was told some thick, nasty black charcoal had to get into her stomach. He gave her a choice of either having a large tube stuck into her nose extending down into her stomach, or drinking it from a glass. Of course she chose the latter.

The lecture was something like this: Whenever a person took more than the prescribed dose of medicine, he or she had lost all basic rights. It was up to the doctor, and only him, to decide what must be done to protect the life of that person. No one could change that order, even if it meant having to strap the person to a bed and force the tube into the stomach, wash it out, then put the charcoal down and admit the patient to the hospital. It was the call of the doctor. It was the awesome responsibility of a doctor and he was not going to take any shortcuts to save the life of a person who abuses a drug. She, the family, the law, nobody could change that decision. Tonight she was lucky - she only had to drink charcoal due to the small quantity of drugs consumed.

The horrified patient was scared and ashamed when she came into the ER but now she was crying and sobbing like a small child being scolded by her father. She heard every word of the lecture, as did her father who had arrived and listened from outside the room. Coming into the room, he said nothing, just gave her a hug and observed. She had a blood draw and made lots of funny faces drinking the activated charcoal. She made promises to her father to never take drugs again.

As assumed, the acetaminophen level was not dangerous after the four-hour blood test. At discharge, she went to the doctor and said a sincere thank-you. Later the doctor said to the staff, "I have given that lecture hundreds of times and this is the first person that cried that hard - it may have done some good this time".

****

A very obese 71 year-old woman was taking a sedative. In the past week she had been having a lot of trouble sleeping even if she took 2 or 3 or 4 pills. She was upset that they did not work and decided to take the rest of the prescription – 9 pills.

Early one evening her daughter found her sleeping, over 18 hours from the time of taking the pills. In other words, they did work. She was still drowsy and drifting off to sleep after being brought into the ER. She comically slurred her attempts to talk, sounding like being under water. Everyone, including her daughter, would smile and giggle which she would recognize as such and point with her own smile. After many trial conversations the complete information was pieced together and details were obtained.

She did need to 'sleep' this off, but with a heart monitor and frequent observations. She was admitted, with fast flowing IV fluids and a foley catheter to drain her bladder and flush out her system. She was still making contortions of her mouth in attempts to talk when she was wheeled upstairs. The family doctor probably will not be prescribing that drug to her again.

****

A good-looking gal of only 50 years was properly dressed in a matching long dress and long sleeved blouse except where the sleeve was cut open to allow the paramedic access for an IV. Her social status would be a prim and proper lady in most circles of society. The EMT reported in route to the ER that she'd had a seizure. On arrival her condition was conscious and alert.

She readily admitted she was an IV drug addict for over 20 years. She pulled up her remaining long sleeve and showed the needle marks of multiple uses. Money was no problem for her, which gave her an excuse. "It is ok if you don't have to get the money illegally to support the habit." Her drug of choice was a powerful, slow–release narcotic pill. Her method was to crush the pills, mix the powder with water, and inject the solution directly into a vein. This is a very dangerous practice, since 12 hours of the narcotic enters the blood stream all at once.

Tonight, she had hit bottom, as many addicts must experience before they get serious about quitting. She took the "hit" and shortly had a full-blown seizure just as her grown daughter arrived at the house. When the seizure was over, she had a sleepy period while the daughter called 911.

Lots of conversations were taking place between her and the staff, doctors, and clergy during her 8 hours of observation in the ER. She admitted she needed to quit and this was the time. She was admitted to the hospital and later transferred to a rehab institute as she had been so many times in the past. According to her, this time would be different.

Two years later, she returned to the ER as a visitor to show that she had been clean since that terrible night. It made us all feel good to know that sometimes, we win. It makes all the stress worth it.

****

Was this man standing in triage as old as he appeared? Was he a true "hillbilly"? He wore stained bib overalls, wading boots, and a torn checkered shirt. Nearby, his wife was chewing on something, slouched over in a dirty sack dress. If the color of her teeth were any indication, tobacco would be assumed.

When asked what was bothering the nervous-acting patient, the answer was a vague, "I have been sick for the past 3 days." He was asked what medications he took. His wife produced a leather pouch with a leather drawstring around the top, containing three bottles of pills.

One was for the heart, and another, an antidepressant. The empty one was a "nerve pill". When asked if he took them for depression he said, "I take 2 kinds of pills to make me feel better." It seems he had been out of that other kind of 'feel good' pill, a nerve pill, for the past 3 days.

He was assigned to an exam room for the doctor to decide what might be done to make this old man "feel better". He was 48 years old and did live in a less inhabited area of the hills. In the end, he was given only 3 more of the missing "nerve" pills and told to see his regular doctor as soon as possible.

After discharge, security personnel came in telling us the story of their vehicle. It was a very old pick up truck with a dead battery and rust all around the body. The interior was shabby, with seat springs popping thru, but protected by a couple of boards. After a jump-start, the engine ran very rough but did make it out of the parking lot. We hoped they made it home to "them thar hills."

****

An older teenager good-looking and clean-cut came in complaining of pain in the bend of his left arm. It was red, swollen and warm. Crying either for the sake of the pain or because his mother was ready to beat him made the events of what happened next more difficult. It was important because it was obviously an infection of the skin, but what ingredient caused it would be important to the kind of treatment.

He had been at a party 3 days ago and wanted to try a "new" high. An accomplice had attempted to inject cocaine into the vein. He admitted he had ingested it before by snorting, but never before injected anything into the vein. The "pusher" missed the vein and put the poison into the tissue under the skin. He said it burned like a hot poker but he thought that must be part of the process of getting a high.

Whining and crying was off and on in the room, but when taken to x-ray he did not utter any sounds. His mother stayed in the room and asked what she should do. She was advised to go home because all the crying and whining was for the purpose of playing to her sympathies. She understood, and as soon as he came back she said goodbye. The young, pitiful-acting patient became quiet and cooperative as soon as she was out of sight.

During the process of getting the IV started in his right arm, he objected because he was "scared of needles". He did not think of that a few days ago, when the needle was put into his arm incorrectly. He was admitted to the hospital for further treatments. This drug attempt was probably the best thing to happen to him , because he said, "I will never let an illegal drug be put into this body again – no matter what the method." During his overnight stay in the hospital, he got antibiotics for the infection called cellulitis. After discharge, he continued with treatments as an outpatient.

$$*********************$$

There are some terms used in private conversations in the ER not intended for the patients that convey the status of a patient. A 70 year-old woman had many of those names attached to her. "Whiner" and "Drug Seeker" were the most understood. Another one was "GOMER", an acronym for 'Get out of my ER". Every time she came in, mostly by ambulance, it was for something so painful normal pain meds would not work. She would whine and look more pitiful than a scolded dog. Even if we chewed her out, she would reply between whines, "God bless you".

It was also known that she took in vagrants of all ages to her filthy home "because they are so needy". Many times she would come to the ER saying her "guest" had stolen her pain pills and left town. Also, she would say they stole her money, so she could not pay for any new pain pills. She was a mess, which added more non-repeatable acronyms.

This 'GOMER' visit was for a twisted ankle that hurt "more then when I had my heart attack". There was no bruising, but there were "tender spots" on every square inch from the knee down to the toe. She requested a cast and a walker plus a powerful narcotic pill by name.

All of the whining and begging requests fell on deaf ears when the x-ray was negative. She was offered some Motrin or Tylenol. This stopped her whining, with an attitude change of 180 degrees producing an irate voiced, angry woman. She jumped off the cot and stomped out of the ER not limping on that leg at all. She was "cured!"

****

A woman came rushing into the ER saying her 21 year-old daughter was having seizures in a car in the ambulance bay. The daughter had premature wrinkles on her face and was literally skin and bones . When she was placed into a wheelchair she denied having a seizure as her mother had said, telling us she was having a narcotic withdrawal. She said her mother was embarrassed to say she was addicted to pain drugs and used the term "seizure" as an excuse.

The patient said she had an appointment with a drug counselor in a few days to get assistance to stop the narcotic obsession. In the meantime, she was "getting a head start" by stopping all drugs cold turkey, which resulted in a withdrawal syndrome. She stated, "I threw all the pills I had into the toilet and flushed them three days ago."

We explained to this pitiful looking patient rolling on the cot groaning in agony that the best way to come clean is to taper off under the direction of a doctor. Her mother was present and seemed to be just as ignorant. The claimed appointment with the counselor was confirmed, so a dose of Valium plus a prescription for more was given to help the patient until she could see the counselor.

In about a half hour the patient was calm and drifting off to sleep as she was "poured" into the back seat of their car. Her mother said she would have help at home to get her into bed. Since the gal was only about 90 pounds it should not have been difficult.

****

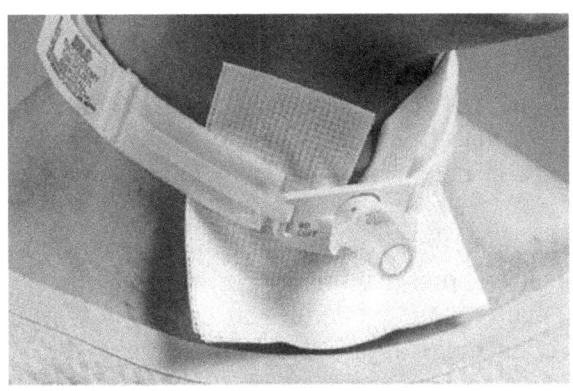

ODDS and ENDS

Most ER cases are emergencies, or at least perceived emergencies. By definition, a medical emergency is a threat of loss of life, or limb, or body function, like a deep laceration or head injury. A major medical emergency would be a true threat of loss of life, like a gunshot, heart attack, automobile accident victim, and so forth.

Other cases are emergencies to the patient like the acute pain of a kidney stone or smashed finger. But the majority of cases seen hour after hour could easily be taken care of in a doctor's office or a fast track clinic. Other times, just a simple over the counter medication would do the trick.

The last type of "emergency" might be cured by the old saying, "time heals all wounds." These include earaches, sore throats, and coughs. Pain that sometimes has persisted for days, weeks, and even months should not be seen in the ER. A doctor, a physician's assistant, or nurse practitioner when over the counter medications fail should see this.

****

A husky 26 year-old male came into the ER complaining of back pain, bending forward with each step. His injury appeared to be a muscle spasm, caused by lifting a riding lawnmower to facilitate fixing a flat tire.

He thought something worse had occurred, but since it happened at 3PM and it was now 8PM his concern was really not justified. He had not taken any medications during this period of time but he did finish fixing the flat tire. When asked why no pain medicine had been taken, his reply was that it might be the wrong thing to do.

A non-narcotic injection for the pain was given, plus a muscle relaxer medication prescription.   He thought he needed more powerful medications, but since he was driving it was not permitted to give a narcotic medication. He left unhappy, the normal result when it turns out a perceived emergency was not the case. He could also have been embarrassed, and mad at himself for the whole situation. Yelling at the ER staff was just a convenient outlet.

****

A 25 year-old gal camping out in a tent had spent most of the day at a theme park in the rain. She looked like an adventurous lady in her cowboy boots with leotards extending from her shorts, topped off with a shirt sporting fringes of beaded strings. She came into the ER with a cough that produced no phlegm, having chills and a sore chest, most likely from the forceful coughing. She had not taken any medication, or even tried to get any.

She said she had no idea what kind of medication she would need even if she had gone to a local drug store. When asked the worst symptom that brought her into the ER, the answer was the cough. Why then, we, asked, would you not go to a local drug store and find a cough medicine? She just shrugged her shoulders.

Her visit included an expensive chest x-ray, blood work, and EKG for the chest pain. The cost would be from $2000 to $3000, resulting in cough medicine and Tylenol. She was given a dose of a cough medication and instructed to get some more over the counter. The drug store visit would have only cost about $5 to $10. She was unhappy, but her cough was better at discharge.

****

Five days had passed since a family outing when a healthy 35 year-old gal came in with knee and chest aches. She was of average weight and build, with a bright smile that warmed the heart of each staff member.

It was determined quickly the chest aches were not cardiac related, since it was made worse when she moved her upper body and her arms. Its' cause was sore muscles, due to the excess activity like baseball and tug of war at the reunion. The fact that she had participated in everything possible made her start to realize she probably had over done it.

She first felt the knee pain as she rounded third base full speed, causing a limp as she continued to run. When asked if she scored a run she hung her head admitting she had to slow down due to the pain, and resulted in being out at home plate. From her story, it appeared she had a high pain tolerance but her grimaces did get the attention of the ER doctor.

3 days before she had gone to her family doctor who did a physical exam, but did not order an x-ray. His professional opinion, per the patient's interpretation, was a possible burst blood vessel within the joint. His theory was that it should get better after the bleeding stopped and the blood was reabsorbed. Feeling no better after 3 more days, she wanted a second opinion, the reason for her visit to the hospital.

In the ER it was noted that as the knee was bent in various positions it was very painful, as the patient's forceful verbal expletives reminded the doctor. Second thoughts were made as to her pain tolerance. An x-ray did not show any bone defects so the diagnosis concluded it was a torn cartilage. Her only comment was that if it hurt that much something should show up.

She left happy, with a knee brace and medications for pain and inflammation. These would also help her muscle aches in the chest.

****

Should a weeklong pain in the left lower abdomen that comes and goes be considered an emergency? A 40 year-old male with excess stomach fat thought so, and came to the ER. His reason was strictly the pain, fearing it "might be appendicitis". He did not know the appendix was on the right side. He admitted he was ignorant of body parts and how they work.

He said his bowel movements were normal the past few days. After x-rays did not show an obstruction or other possible problems, it was determined he had diverticulitis, an inflammation of the colon.

He was put on antibiotics and good pain pills and referred to a gastroenterologist. He laughed like a jello-bellied Santa while asking, "Is that all there is to the pain I have been having?" Little did he know that appendicitis was a much simpler, easier, and quicker problem to overcome. He now had a lifetime problem, but his next doctor will tell him that.

****

A lady looked older then the 58 years that appeared on her paperwork. Her hair was uncombed, with strands sticking out all over as if she had put a finger in a light socket. She wore no makeup and sported wrinkled clothes with mismatched socks completing the package. Soft-spoken words in a monotone flow indicated a touch of depression.

She had been fighting pneumonia for 10 days, with coughing that would not let her sleep. She had just completed a course of antibiotics and steroids but the cough was so bad she would gag and then have heaving spells. "Completely worn out" were the words, which her appearance confirmed. She did say her breathing was somewhat better than before.

The routine tests and x-rays were completed, resulting in a diagnosis of bronchitis. The previous treatment corrected the pneumonia but the irritation in her windpipe was now the new complication. A strong cough syrup was given, plus another type of antibiotic.

Following discharge, she stayed for an extra half hour in the waiting room, to see if the coughing was helped. Before she left, she returned to the doctor and gave him a big hug and a smile. This was repeated with every nurse the jubilant lady came to, plus the cleaning person mopping the floor. The reason was because she had not coughed for 15 minutes. She was happy, and even took time to wash her face and run her fingers thru her hair. She looked years younger.

****

She looked like a stick figure being wheeled into the ER by a friend. A large plastic pan was in her lap with her head hanging low, allowing her hair to almost touch its' ugly contents. She was 5 foot 4 inches and weighed only 82 pounds on her 78 year-old frame.

Her companion stated that long ago she weighed 150 pounds, but in the past 5 years had suffered severe depression. This caused her loss of appetite.

Nausea with vomiting for days was the reason for her ER visit. Earlier in the week her doctor had prescribed anti-nausea suppositories but they had failed to work. She continued to have nausea with dry heaves, especially if she tried to eat or drink. Her abdomen was caved inward to the degree the back bone might be visible.

IV fluids with anti-nausea medication were infused over the next two hours. Toward the end of the last hour she stated nausea was gone and wanted a drink of water. We explained a drink at this moment would start the nausea and vomiting all over again, but she insisted on a drink. Even though a sip was encouraged, she took a big gulp. With anxious anticipation all present waited for the gagging, heaving, and vomiting to start. Nothing happened. What a relief for her and everyone else!

The patient raised her head just enough to see her face, revealing a hint of a grin. She was admitted into the hospital for observation and nutrition. Hopefully help with depression would be included.

In some ways this was an emergency, but a return visit to her doctor might have resulted in an admission to the hospital also.

****

The dance of the sobbing gal coming down the hall was all too familiar to most. Her torso was gyrating like a rock and roller adding a lateral move to keep the virtual hula-hoop going around. Both hands were held tightly against the lower left side of her body. Her feet would step wide, then narrow, and finally cross over the other, making the entire width of the hallway her dance floor.

It was known to most as "the kidney stone dance". The 30 year-old gal had never had this much pain, even with childbirth. She said she had vomited just before coming into the ER. The gyration continued while the IV was attempted three times. She forced a quiet moment the fourth time and the needle did not "jump" out of place before it was secured with lots of tape.

For a period of time, maybe half an hour, this gal was crying and muffling her screams when the medications were given and she was taken to the cat scan. About the time they were ready to scan she stopped all sounds causing the technician to think she had passed out, or died. She suddenly started laughing loudly proclaiming the pain was all gone. The scan was completed and did not show a kidney stone.

Smiles, glee, and relief were in abundance when she returned to the ER room. Her husband was dumbfounded. It was explained to them that the stone probably moved into the bladder and no longer was scratching the walls of the ureter. Instructions were given to strain all urine to catch the stone to be analyzed. Her curt reply was, "I ain't catching anything. I don't want that thing, let it get flushed away."

****

A 45 year-old man was at a party of mixed couples complete with a lot of mixed drinks. He was not inhibited in trying to compliment a lady by making reference to her upper anatomy. The husband was within hearing and had uninhibited jealousy, resulting in a blow to the man's temple with a beer bottle. A witness relayed the story adding the man was dazed but did not fall down. About 15 minutes later he staggered and fell onto the couch.

When EMS arrived, they saw a drunken guest performing CPR on the downed man saying with a slurred voice, "He 'sopped' livin so I do it fer em." A sore chest was the only thing that came of the efforts of that "rescuer" since his heart rate was normal.

On arrival to the ER he had short periods of combative behavior and slurred speech with continuous nausea, but no vomiting. He constantly was asking for the lady at the party to apologize for what he said. He complained of a headache and some blurred vision. All this meant a stat cat scan of the brain.

The blow to his temple region had been strong enough to cause bleeding in his brain called a "sub-arachnoid bleed". This was a true emergency needing to be in the trauma room and not in the non-emergency section.

About 30 minutes later he was in a helicopter to another facility with a neurosurgeon. The odds were slim of him making it, but a report the next day said he was going to make it but may have some mental deficits.

92

****

A dilemma for a 61 year-old gentleman who recently had colon resection surgery happened as the patient was brought into the empty ER at 4AM. The IV for this procedure had been in his right wrist and it was removed when he was discharged. In the meantime that site had gotten infected with redness, hot skin, and pain up to the elbow. It is called phlebitis and must be corrected with antibiotics before it spreads into the blood stream.

This man said he was a reasonable person afraid of needles, but when it caused problems he did not want anything to do with another one. Another IV had to be started to give him the proper care. A lot of people and a lot of reasoning were provided and he finally gave in and permitted the IV in the other arm. Once it was in place he relaxed, stating he knew it had to be done but was hoping for an alternative.

He returned to the ER four more times for an antibiotic infusion using the same IV each time. The redness and pain subsided a lot by the end of the 5th infusion and he was then put on pills for 10 days. When the IV was removed after that 5th time, he was told no promises, but an infection was not the plan. He had a sheepish grin upon hearing that plan, telling us he was still afraid of needles!

****

A female friend brought in a 30 year-old, 240-pound man who told this story of how he dislocated his shoulder: "I was getting dressed, pulling up my pants. I didn't know that the leg of the pants was caught on the bed - I thought I was standing on them. I got mad, jumped up off the floor and yanked on the pants as hard as I could. The pain in my shoulder was so intense I fell to the floor."

Being a muscular person (or as one female nurse stated, 'no parts wasted on fat') the spasms of the shoulder were in full force. It took lots of morphine and Valium to relax him enough to forcefully pull the arm bone back into place. Due to the large amount of medicine, he was humorous for the next few hours with slurred speech, unreasonable requests, and more statements that would embarrass even him if he heard them.

The question remains as to why this person was pulling on his pants at 2AM. We never did ask if it happened at home. The female friend had left long ago.

****

The right wrist of a 58 year-old female was infected from a two-day-old surgical procedure. She was beside herself because of the chest pain it was causing. Sounded crazy, but other details were needed. She was a slim gal with normally fair skin, but now was red from local fever. Her husband stated she was normally reserved and quiet, but she could not understand what was happening and became hysterical at times.

She had a mastectomy on the right side 1 year ago. She pulled back her blouse and revealed that the right side of her chest formerly occupied by a breast was inflamed and swollen to almost a fourth the size of her remaining left breast. It was also very tender and she would not let her clothing touch that side. She added it would be nice to replace the missing breast, but not this way.

She was informed that mastectomy also involved removing the lymph nodes in the underarm area, and her body was having difficulty dealing with the new infection in the wrist. This caused the lymph nodes in her chest to take over and swell, called lymphedema.

After doses of 2 different antibiotics, an anti-inflammatory, and pain meds she calmed down and promised to get to her surgeon the next day. She also promised her husband she would not have to get hysterical now that she knew what was happening. He seemed to relax a little.

****

"I just about passed out, but now I am just fine" were the opening words from a 70 year-old man as he walked into the ER. He stated that as the church service was starting, he was standing for a long time during the opening songs. He suddenly got dizzy and had to sit for about 10 minutes. When he was no longer dizzy but felt weak, he and his wife left the church. Saying nothing to him, his wife drove directly to the ER insisting he get checked. He came in objecting to such nonsense.

All tests for near syncope (passing out) were negative. He turned to his wife with the 'I told you so' look. She smiled and said she wanted to be sure. The doctor surmised aloud to them that he had probably locked his knees back while standing, causing pooling of blood in the lower legs resulting in less blood to the brain, and that can make anyone pass out, or at least get dizzy.

It was the wife's turn to give that 'look' and say, " I told you it was all your doing to get out of going to church."

****

One summer morning two Jehovah Witness men made a visit to a home where a sloppily dressed, unshaven 70 year-old man answered the door. They determined something must be wrong, and since he lived by himself there was no one with whom they could check. The man did ramble his sentences, and seemed a little unsteady on his feet. He could answer their questions only after a long pause, as if to absorb the question or conjure up an answer, or both.

A call was made to 911. When the ambulance arrived, the man's son (who lived next door,) came to see what all the commotion was about. He determined his father was not acting any different than any other day. The pair of men insisted medical help was needed and the son argued only a short time, thinking maybe he was missing something.

Of course all tests came back negative except his anti-seizure medication level, which was slightly low. It was learned he had not forgotten to take his medicines that morning. The son had an 'I told you so' attitude as the missionaries apologized. After an extra dose of medication the rambling and hesitant replies improved. The patient seemed to pull himself together asking, "Where am I?"

****

Why was an 86 year-old woman in the ER at 3 AM with a four-day-old "off and on" right side pain? She had a gruff voice with short staccato sentences brought on by the pain to breathe. She arrived by car in a dirty gown, torn ragged along the hem. The sagging skin on her plump cheeks formed jowls like a bulldog. She demanded some pain relief every time she had to move.

The symptoms during assessment indicated a muscular, skeletal origin instead of an ailment of the kidney, liver, gallbladder or lung. The doctor ordered a dose of narcotic pain medication higher then normal for her age. The explanation was "If she wants pain relief so bad she will get it." In a few minutes she was pain free slurring her speech to the point of no understanding.

All tests were negative but she could not be discharged until the narcotic wore off to a safe level. At her age the metabolism is slow, and takes a long time. She stayed in the ER under the watchful eyes of the staff for six hours before her neighbor was called to come get her. She was still talking silly when she was 'poured' into the car.

****

An 18 year-old high school dropout had been married, divorced, and was now living with her new boyfriend when she came into the ER with "severe" groin pain. She was diagnosed with both a urinary tract infection and pelvic inflammatory disease. One of the instructions at discharge was no sex until this was all cleared up, as much as 2 weeks. The look on her face and her boyfriend's face was precious. That was so mean, but totally necessary.

****

It was a slow night in the ER giving the opportunity for staff members to sit and visit. A continuous round table of past experience stories went on for over an hour. Most of the time the present "tale of the past" was an attempt to top the previous. The more gross and the more gruesome the details, the more it was enjoyed. A veteran female nurse had the winner - and she swears it was absolutely true.

She was a student nurse "way back" when she had a respiratory patient who had a tube inserted into his throat for breathing, called a tracheotomy. From time to time mucous globs, called "honkers", had to be cleared from the inside of the bronchi that go to the lungs. The procedure was a squirt of normal saline water in the tracheotomy to loosen the glob and then suction it out. The nurse stated she was new to the event, and each time it was disgusting and almost made her sick. Every 4 hours she had to go into this patient's room to get his "honker".

Some people who have had these devices for a long time get good at expelling a "honker" by blowing it out the tracheotomy after the water treatment. On one of the treatment sessions, an experienced respiratory therapist went in with her. The squirt of water went into the extended tube from the hole in his throat. Next he pulled out a 12" diameter plastic bulls-eye and taped it onto the TV screen. The patient suddenly took a slow, deep breath, aimed the tube extension, and with a huge puff blew air out his trach. The sticky, yellow-colored piece of slime flew out and hit the bulls-eye.

The son sitting nearby congratulated the father, "Good shot". The patient gave an "AAaahhhh" of relief. The respiratory therapist gave a cheer. The storyteller said with a look of guilt, "I passed out".

PS - No one could top that one - so the stories were suspended for the night, allowing some paperwork to get done.

****

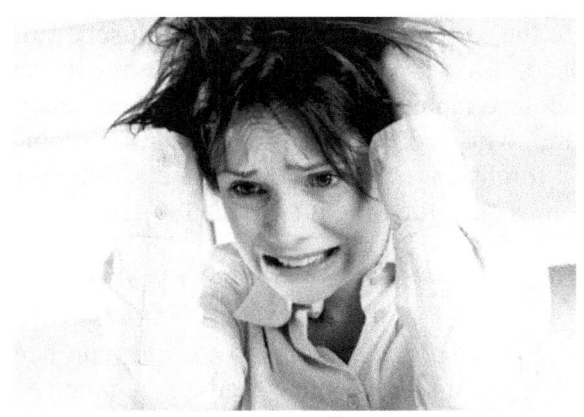

ANXIETY

Anxiety and panic attacks are considered more prevalent in females and teens. Most of the time it is hyperventilation requiring someone to talk them down to a normal breathing pattern. The more pronounced ones are usually middle aged and older adults with a history of panic attacks. The true panic attack presents with nausea, flushed or pale face, profuse sweating, gasping for breath, a scared look in the eyes, and once in a while, a hallucination. Treatment is calming the patient down, and many times a medication to calm the nerves.

****

"It feels like my heart is trying to jump out of my chest," proclaimed a gray haired 60 year-old lady as she was put in the ER room. "It makes me think I just ran a marathon the way my heart is racing." She sat down on the cot clutching her chest as if to hold everything inside. Her eyes were full of fear and her mouth was wide open, even when she was not talking. Panic attacks had been common years ago, but not recently.

Her pulse was high with an elevated blood pressure even though her blood pressure medicine had been taken shortly before arrival. Additional blood pressure reducing meds were given. A few hours later she did feel better with a slower pulse rate and a normal to low blood pressure for her age.

She was well dressed but her makeup was streaked down her

face due to the earlier sweats that were profusely running down from her forehead. One of the techs gave her a mirror so she could "fix her face" before facing the public. She looked better as she left with her husband, who had remained in the waiting room the whole time. He said "I might have had my own panic attack if I had to listen to her any longer than the time it took me to get her here.

****

Four years previously a 36 year-old man had a heart attack, requiring bypass surgery. Since then he frequently came to the ER with "chest pain" and this visit was the second time in one week. His call light was used frequently in order to have someone figuratively come in to hold his hand even after a full battery of heart related tests came back negative. To add to the situation he was suffering from gout with pain in his great toe.

Suddenly he proclaimed "Oh, No!" followed by a full-blown panic attack such as he was prone to, under stress. He got nauseated, sweating profusely, pale skin, and was saying, "This must be the big one". Literally, holding his hand at this time was necessary, as a repeat heart tracing proved to be negative again. An anti-anxiety med calmed him down and he was admitted for observation. He still was not convinced it had nothing to do with his heart. It must be difficult to live in such fear.

****

A 48 year-old lady never had any major health problems in her life. But this evening she had 2 health events. She had a panic attack when she was told she was being admitted for a possible heart attack. Not that the tests proved it, but the story she told was that earlier it felt like an elephant was sitting on her chest, a classic sign of a heart problem. She could not believe it, and started crying, hyperventilating, and sweating with an increase in pulse and blood pressure. A nerve medication helped calm her down and prevented the "possible" heart attack from occurring, at least on the ER watch.

****

A 62 year-old man was clutching his chest as he got out of

the taxi. He said he had a feeling of pressure in his chest and neck. Anxiety was written all over his face and he kept taking quick looks to the side and behind him while being wheeled to a trauma room. The whole time the IV, oxygen, EKG, vital signs and history were obtained he mentioned repeatedly that his wife was out of town visiting friends. The complete heart workup was negative. High blood pressure medicine was given with some results but a nerve med did calm him down along with the blood pressure.

Anxiety with near panic attack without a cause was the mystery until his daughter came in. She stated he gets these "panic attacks" whenever his wife was gone, or going out of town. She continued by saying he was afraid of being alone and this was how he subconsciously or maybe consciously dealt with the situation. Even though the wife knows it may happen she will leave and stay away so she does not have to deal with it. He was sent home with his daughter.

****

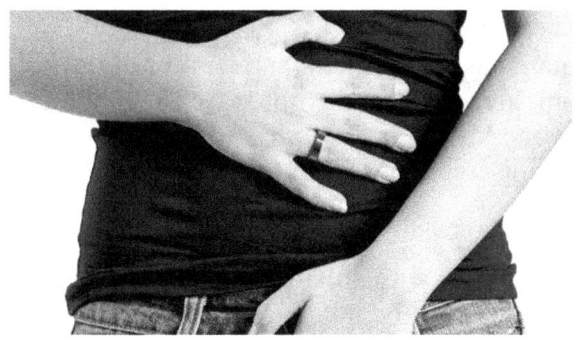

<u>URINARY</u>

Only two cases are presented for memorable patients with urinary problems. Retention, kidney stones, and infections are common. Most of the patients who come into the ER with one of these complications have either had them before or know the details of some friend or relative with the same thing. They know what has to be done and also know things will come out ok. The ones here are typical, but the patient in one reacted more graciously than most and the other one was an unexpected diagnosis to all.

****

"Please help me, I am in so much pain" were the first words a middle aged man said as he entered the triage area of the ER. There was anguish and a hint of tears on his face along with a bent over posture. There was no doubt of his severe pain, confirmed when he said it had been 24 hours since he had gone to the bathroom.

Since urinary retention is a common occurrence, the protocol dictates we get him comfortable as soon as possible. He was taken directly to a room where he told his story the best he could. The stammering words were huffs and puffs of pain-riddled breathing. Quickly a catheter was inserted and relief was immediate as copious amounts of urine output drained into the bag.

"You are an angel that I owe my life", the patient repeated over and over, as his bladder drained 4 times the normal amount. " I want to let everyone know how great a nurse you are, but it might be a little hard to explain why."

The man was now content and could not stop talking. "I live 50 miles from here but would not go to my hometown hospital because everyone knows me and that would be embarrassing. The drive here was miserable but worth it for the fast treatment and great relief."

About a week later a large box of candy arrived in the ER addressed to the nurse, with a thank-you note from the patient about how wonderful it was to be treated with dignity and speed, and get total relief. The entire staff wanted to know the patient's problem, and the nurse refused to say, due to confidentiality laws. It was also against the law for them to look it up on the charts, so it remained a secret from that moment on. Of course, everyone helped devour the sweets in short order.

****

A 45YO gal came into triage during the slower part of the morning (5AM) saying, "Since midnight I've been having pains right here" as she pointed to her lower right side. She looked miserable with drooping eyes, limp hanging arms, and a shuffling walk. She had a history of kidney stones, but she thought this felt more like a urinary tract infection. She did not come in doing the "kidney stone dance" but more the "UTI freeze". The "freeze" would happen when the urinary tract inflammation caused burning with urination. To fight the urge to urinate, the legs were held together until the need to 'go' was lessened.

She was instructed to provide a sample in a little jar. "Please, is there any other way to get the sample? It hurts so bad to go." The answer was a catheter, so there was a grimace and freshened resolve to try the painful way.

When she emerged from the bathroom she had a huge smile. Holding the cup at arm's length she said, "I feel a lot better - look what's in the bottom." There was a tiny speck of a brown kidney stone. It must have passed out of the ureter, into the bladder, and out to the cup all at the same time. She was embarrassed to have held back for so long, but the inner pressure must have helped bring the situation to an end.

The contented and happy patient was ready to go home but had to remain for a lab analysis of the urine to rule out the urinary tract infection.

There was now a spring in her step and a sparkle in her eyes. She was tired from no sleep most of the night, and fell asleep for the hour it took to complete our lab work. Tests were negative for a UTI and she was discharged with the stone in a jar, and a smile on her face.

****

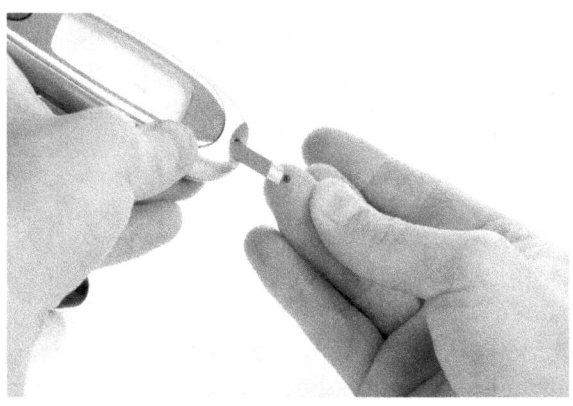

DIABETICS

Diabetes has always been the most common chronic disease. Obesity has been blamed but other factors such as genes have been added to the heredity possibilities. When a diabetic goes off his prescribed diet, pills, or injections to maintain the best glucose level, they become a patient and end up in the ER.

****

A 36 year-old rather slender gal was moved quickly into a trauma room after her blood sugar test was completed. Her diagnosis was acute diabetic ketoacidosis, a reading of 436. Her eyes were drooping as she sat on the edge of the cot breathing rapidly. Having been fighting this breathing pattern for 2 to 3 days made her look like a wet rag flapping in the breeze. Her skin was hot and her breath had a sickly sweet smell. She admitted not taking any of her medicines for the past seven days.

She said, "The medicines are making me fat." She had liposuction and a breast reduction in the past meaning a slim figure was very important to her. When confronted with the option of either life or a good figure she did hesitate before answering. "I would rather be dead than be fat." A silent "wow" echoed in the room.

Insulin IV was slowly administered dropping her blood sugar count to 341, a level ICU would accept for care. During the admit process reminders about the importance of proper medicine were discussed with this good-looking but very sick girl. Her frequent response, "How can I control my weight and still take the medicine?" It always came back to the "fat" in the medicine. Hopefully, some more in-depth education was made available to her during the stay in the hospital.

****

High blood sugar caught the patient off guard. He had called two friends for help and when they arrived at his place he was lying in the front doorway.

Once they arrived at the ER with the 31 year-old patient they reported he was a fragile diabetic. There was a sweet smell of "Karo Syrup" on his breath. The glucose level test of his blood read a near record high of 478, a number only a young person might tolerate.

After 2 hours of slow insulin IV treatment the patient was conscious and able to tell his part of the story. He had started a new job and forgot to take his insulin for at least 2 days. Once he started to feel dizzy and thirsty and had frequent trips to the bathroom he remembered the insulin. He gave himself a shot. He stumbled and crawled to the front door in time to hear a car pull into the driveway. He said he did not recall calling his friends or anything after that until a few moments ago.

His new job was in a donut shop. The consumption of an extra donut or two did not help his condition. He was admitted to continue the slow insulin drip until his blood sugar returned to normal which for him had been 130.

He promised a dozen donuts for the ER when he got back to work, including the two that he would not eat anymore.

****

A lady from out of town was unpacking when she realized she had forgotten her accu-chek machine, the one that measures the glucose level in the blood.

It was after hours and all drug stores were closed, so she and her husband arrived at the ER for a blood sugar check. Her claim was that she needed that number to be able to take the right amount of insulin.

To get a blood glucose check, a doctor's order was required after being checked into the ER. The slightly plump lady stood upright with a smile and said she needed the blood test so check her in. The cost of this visit would buy many machines the next morning.

Another option would have been to drive over 35 miles to a nearby town with an all night drug store. She still had that pleasant smile and rejected the option. The doctor had another option. Why not just take the average insulin injection for this one night. It would not be that far off to cause a problem and she could get a new machine tomorrow morning.

The lady and her husband still insisted they get it checked, and even get the indicated dose of insulin in the ER since it was already past due time for her normal evening dose. The conclusion was that their doctor had done a good education on the importance of calculating the right amount each and every time. Common sense and frugal concepts were thrown out for the sure thing.

****

A middle-aged man was pounding on the door to the ambulance bay. His 55 year-old spouse was slumped over in the front seat of the car, not moving. He said she was diabetic and had not eaten anything that day. He did not know if she had taken any of her diabetic medicine. With little difficulty the nurse and tech took the frail, pale, wrinkle-skinned patient from the car into a wheelchair. A lot of groans and snorts emitted from clenched teeth but her eyes were closed.

When she was put into the trauma room the snoring was quite loud and she did not react to any of the sudden moves or plops onto the cot from the wheelchair. Due to the history by the husband the doctor present made a clinical diagnosis of insulin shock. If no food was ingested and insulin was taken it would drop the blood sugar way below 50, the critical level.

She was limp and did not even change the snoring rhythm sounds when the IV needle was inserted. As quickly as possible, the glucose solution was started and to be infused over a two-minute period. Before the infusion was completed the patient awoke, looked around the room and stared at all the people standing her looking down. In a scared voice, she looked at the cables hooked up to her and asked, "Where in the hell am I?". Then she spotted her husband and asked in a gruff voice, "What in the world is happening?"

The entire staff and husband dropped their shoulders from the tension position to the relaxed position. In a matter of 10 minutes this gal progressed from being unconscious in the car to fully functioning. This medical emergency was and will always be the most dramatic miracle that can happen in the ER.

****

A 31 year-old male who came into the ER because he was having a 'really bad headache.' During the medical history questions he stated he was a diabetic. The normal protocol is to check the blood glucose level, which he said he had checked at home just 6 hours ago with a reading of 230. The readings from the test in ER indicated it was 430.

Just a year ago he had been labeled as fragile diabetic when his blood levels changed rapidly with little medication or food. The previous day he said the reading was 200. He had taken his normal medications since then. He was puzzled, as was the doctor, but a repeat blood test confirmed the dangerously high level. He had even taken his insulin shot 5 hours ago, which should have lowered the glucose instead of allowing it to go higher.

Treatment had to be slow so after 2 hours of ER treatments his number came down to 320 and his headache was better. He was admitted to the hospital for further treatment. Hopefully he will be able to control his blood glucose with a better medication routine. It may be a difficult assignment.

****

He weighed less than 150 pounds and was over 6 foot tall. He looked like a living skeleton placed into a wheelchair from a friend's car. The short ride to the trauma room with this unresponsive 48 year old with his head slumped forward was dramatic, as he moved around like a bobble head. When he was transferred, nearly thrown from the wheelchair to the cot, he started to be combative but quickly subsided to a restless form lying there.

His eye sockets were dark rings of black against the white skin of his cheeks. There was a strong odor of alcohol and stains of bloody emesis on his shirt. A medical necklace stated he was diabetic.

The accu-chek for glucose level stated 'out of range' meaning over 600 with a normal range usually 50 to 100. An IV was established as his friends were explaining the condition of the apartment. Many empty liquor bottles all around, emesis pools in the middle of the room, clothes strewn all around, and no signs of food consumption. They had received a call from him earlier stating he was about to pass out and needed help. He was found lying in the front room near the door.

During the protocol treatments of insulin, IV fluids, and oxygen he suddenly quieted from his restless state. The monitor was showing a heart rate of 120 but his chest was not rising and falling. Assisted breathing and intubation were done. His heart rate started to slow down and soon was near zero when chest compressions were started. We had a full code blue protocol for the next half hour. When no spontaneous heartbeat or breathing could be re-established he was pronounced dead.

It was determined the cause of death was uncontrolled diabetes with acute alcohol poisoning. Lab tests showed an alcohol level near 30% and glucose level of over 1200. Was it suicide?

****

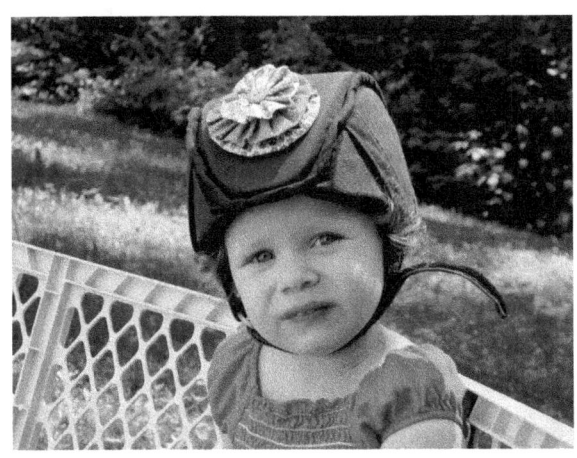

SEIZURE

Is it a seizure if a person is semi-conscious, with twitching and jerking? That is a tough question to answer. Other signs to look for are possible urinary incontinence (peeing), fecal incontinence (bowel movement) and eyes rolling upwards (common). What happens after the twitching stops?

Within the definition of seizure it is stated, "Following a grand-mal seizure, there may be a period of quiet dream-like sleep or continued semi-consciousness." Like fingerprints, no two seizures are alike. Most memorable cases involve some level of misinterpretation of the witnessed signs.

As an example, the mother of a 4 year-old girl said her daughter's daily seizures were too numerous to count. After observing the patient in the ER, the mother suddenly yelled, "There is one now!" Everyone present was looking at the sleeping child and no one saw anything unusual. The mother explained there was a twitch of the hand. In other words, she had become so obsessed with her daughter's diagnosed seizure condition that her definition was way out of proportion. Most everybody who has ever watched a child sleeping will notice jerks of some part of the body. If more than one jerk occurs, the comment is usually, 'She must be dreaming'. Therefore, witnessed accounts of a "seizure" must include details of exactly what they saw.

However, if the patient arrives in the ER semi-conscious,

with wet pants combined with a bitten lower lip and the witness says it was a seizure, we would conclude it was a "tonic/clonic grand-mal seizure".

There is no blood test that can be done for the diagnosis of a seizure. The only thing to do in the ER is rule out other possibilities such as brain bleed, tumor, or other physical findings that would cause similar signs.

****

"There were sixteen (16) seizures in 3 hours". That was the report given to the ambulance EMTs from the mother of a 45 year-old man. He was alert with dry pants. Since being a teenager this 300-pound man had lived with an epileptic seizure disorder and currently took 3 different kinds of medicine for control. Records did show six times in the past year he had come to the ER following a seizure.

The ambulance report added he had not had any more seizures during the trip to the ER. The mother claimed the EMTs did not know what to look for, as he surely must have had more. She came by car with the patient's wife. The doctor wanted the man's wife to go into detail about what had happened during the past 3 hours. She had a calm voice, with a "matter of fact" experienced method of telling the story in detail. She seemed well educated about her husband's disorder, using all the proper terminology such as "grand-mal", petite mal, postictal, and more. Her clothing was clean with an ironed look and her reddish hair was mostly in place. She quickly volunteered with a look of pride that she had Down's Syndrome and was the main caregiver to her disabled husband. She mesmerized the staff with her presentation, since her features were mongoloid but did not show the usual mannerisms associated with Downs.

She said, "In the beginning his body got tense, with some jerking, and his eyes were closed for about 1 minute. The rest of the 15 times consisted of twitching of fingers and hands with his eyes rolling upward, lasting about 10 seconds each over a 3 hour period. He was able to communicate well after each episode".

Between the patient and his wife a good history was obtained, with small additions of "clarity" from his mother. Our impression was that the patient and his wife did not consider the little ones as "seizures".

It was the mother-in-law who did the counting during those 3 hours, and she had been the one who called 911, accounting for the high number reported from the start. They did not want to upset the mother by disagreeing at this time.

In the end a blood test did show a slightly low level of anti-seizure meds, and more was given by IV after a consult with his neurologist. He had no seizure-like episodes in the ER and was discharged after a few hours. Throughout the rest of the evening lots of comments were made by the ER staff about the remarkable woman who had overcome her Down's Syndrome.

****

For the past 4 years a 19 year-old gal had a history of "syncopal episodes" or passing out, but no twitching or jerking. In the beginning, it was blamed on a "teenager thing". Now she had been married for 3 months and was on a honeymoon accompanied by both her mother and mother-in-law.

She had never been diagnosed in the past as having seizures, which was good since it would follow her the rest of her life even if it were proved she was not having an actual seizure. She took no seizure preventing medications. She was good looking and a little plump, but she carried it well. Her blond hair was flowing half way down her back, and she liked to toss her head to make the hair fly.

She arrived by wheelchair through the ER doors, with her husband pushing and the two mothers following. She was alert and "feeling tired" but her eyes had the appearance of being wide-awake. She quickly got out of the chair, spinning around to sit on the ER cot. A smile came across her face as she said, "You are not going to ruin my honeymoon, are you?" The reply from the quick-witted doctor was, "Not any more than having your mothers along." The mothers laughed.

****

Sitting in a recliner earlier at the motel she had a "passing out" event. The husband and mothers said there was some jerking of her arms during the time she was out.

It was less then a minute and she awoke not remembering the

event. Because she felt tired they allowed her to sit there for about half an hour before deciding to bring her to the ER when she did not get better.

It was usually not the ER doctor's place to write a diagnosis of "seizure" with a first time event not witnessed by trained medical members. She passed all the tests to rule out other possible causes. Her discharge "suggestions" were "do not do anything dangerous (like tightrope walking) or driving until cleared by her doctor or neurologist." The cause might have been stress related since her new husband was also getting chemotherapy for a lymphoma. Adding that to a wedding, honeymoon, and both mothers made for "extraordinary stress".

She was told to continue her honeymoon with another diagnosis of "syncopal episode". Since she knew all the negative ramifications of a "seizure diagnosis" she left saying, "This place is the most understanding of all the other medical places I have been." She was an admirable and memorable woman.

****

A 57 year-old man was attending a live music show. At intermission he stood up, and seemed to pass out into the arms of another man who helped him to the floor. His wife and others told the EMTs they witnessed him having jerks of his limbs, but his eyes were closed so they could not tell if his eyes rolled. About 1 minute later he stopped all movements, opened his eyes, and wanted to know what happened. The people around him said he'd had a seizure and repeated this to the EMTs. He and his wife said he had no history of seizures.

Upon arriving at the ER, the patient was alert with no indications of incontinence. He said, "I am feeling great and just want to go home." He appeared an average person, not overweight, and sat upright in anticipation of the next question.

His occupation was an over the road truck driver, and a seizure diagnosis would be devastating. With a flip of his head and hand he surmised, "This probably is a result of going to 3 or 4 shows per day on a bus tour for the past week and I am just worn out." .

Did he have a seizure, or did he just pass out by standing up suddenly? All tests to rule out other causes were negative. His only current condition included colon surgery for cancer and he had a temporary colostomy bag, plus diet controlled diabetes.

In the end, a diagnosis of "syncopal-episode" (passing out) was made with a verbal condition. He was not to drive a car until a neurologist cleared him when he got home. If a similar event happened while driving, the consequences could be serious. He reluctantly accepted the diagnosis and conditions adding, "The bus driver will do all the driving to get me home." He also was advised to not stand up quickly, just in case. His parting comment, "The music show was not all that great anyway."

****

Was it a seizure, drug related reactions, or something else? These were our questions after hearing the ambulance report of a 28 year-old having a seizure. The facts did not add up, and the first test (urine for drugs) did reveal marijuana and benzodiazepine (Valium like) substances in his system, but not enough to be of concern.

The patient got home and his mother stated that he was not acting right. He started to hallucinate, saying his brother was chasing him and wanted to kill him. At the same time, he told his mother he had a headache. He fell to the floor and all limbs started to jerk violently, giving his mother the idea of a seizure. A few minutes later he started to yell about the same hallucination, but had no more jerking.

EMS stated he kept yelling most of the trip to the ER and then "passed out". He was of average height and weight with bruises showing around his left eye, and more injury marks on his shoulder and the underside of both forearms. They were in a defensive pattern, seen when a victim held his arms in front of his face while being hit.

A cat scan indicated a possible concussion and hematoma (blood clot) on the brain. His brother arrived, relaying the story from one week ago. The patient had been in a brawl and gotten kicked in the head numerous times. He had a terrible headache afterwards, but refused to report it or get medical help because he did not have any money or insurance. During the next week, he slept most of the time at his brother's apartment.

The brain damage from the fight could have caused his actions that evening and may have been the reason for the seizure.

He needed further evaluations and care in another hospital. He was transferred as a concussion patient but not as a seizure patient. If he had gotten immediate help the story might have had a better ending. The whole case was a shame.

****

After five years of taking seizure prevention medications, a 27 year-old woman's doctor took her off all of them because she was 4 months pregnant. She was told this might lessen possible complications from the medications. The seizures had started after a serious accident with a concussion. The number of seizures since then was minimal and there had been none for the past year.

She went to a local Christmas tree lighting ceremony and all the lights on the tree came on at once, with strobe lights flashing repeatedly. At that moment, she grabbed her husband and started shaking like a leaf. He put her on the ground and let the jerking and frothing at the mouth subside. He said it lasted about 3 minutes in total. There had been one more similar seizure in the ambulance.

In the ER, she admitted she not only had incontinence of urine but of the bowels also. It had been over a half hour since the event, her sleepy state was almost over, and she could communicate clearly. She said she felt tired with no headache. All the normal tests were good.

She was administered some anti-seizure medication by IV and admitted to the hospital for further evaluation of the fetus. She said, I can feel movement from the baby," which was good, plus the fetal heart tones were strong. She should be able to complete her pregnancy and have a good life but would have to keep taking at least a small dose of medications to prevent another seizure. There was one added directive, not to attend functions with strobe lights.

****

A 38 year-old gal with frequent seizures for the past three years following a head injury accident had most unusual movements during her seizures. She would not jerk, flail, or even twitch her

arms and legs, but would just rigidly arch her back. "I guess it is from my desire to be a contortionist," she said with a smile.

One event in the ER was very impressive because the top of her head and bottoms of her feet were on the bed, but the middle of her back was at least 2 feet off the bed. She rigidly held that position a full 2 minutes and then collapsed in a semi-sleep. Her family said that was normal for her.

After a few hours of medication she was not having any more events. Her neurologist was contacted and he ordered a different medication than what had been given. The process of changing over to the new medication took a long time, since adding the two together may have been too much for her system to handle. Five hours later the new medication was on board and she was alert and ready to be admitted into the hospital. That was when she started to complain of a headache.

She placed the back of her hand on her forehead when the nurse got close to her face. Suddenly the patient flung her arm out straight, striking the nurse in the chest and knocking her back into the wall. The arch of the patient's back happened quickly and lasted for a few minutes.

A dose of the first medication was quickly given. It seemed the original drug was not going to work. Close observation of her vital signs was now a must because the two meds had to be given closer together than medically recommended.

Moments later she fell down onto the bed and went into a deep sleep, to the extent that only the heart monitor was indicating she was still alive and blood oxygen level was satisfactory. She was admitted to ICU where it would now be their problem.

****

A 32 year-old portly man with cerebral palsy had mild seizures up to 6 times per day. His various caregivers, both live- in and hired, were familiar to these episodes, making sure he did not hurt himself. He had severe allergic reactions to every kind of anti-seizure medication tried. Some even caused anaphylactic shock and cessation of breathing. There were about 12 different pills he took to help control the episodes and the palsy.

On rare occasions he had a grand mal seizure, with flailing arms and feet. His caregivers could not deal with those, and usually called the ambulance. In the ER there was not much that could be done except give him comfort without medications. It surely was not the way to live. He was admitted for observation and maybe a change in some of those 12 pills taken daily.

****

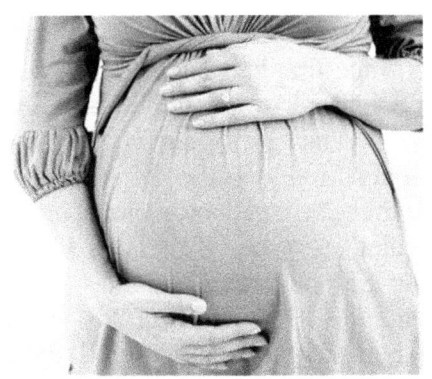

PREGNANCY

Pregnancy emergencies are rare in the ER. Most of the time the perceived emergencies are just uninformed mothers and fathers supposing the tiny fetus is in trouble. It can be strange or new pains; not feeling the baby move; vaginal spotting; and other minor but normal events that happen during the 9 months. True emergencies like stillbirths, premature delivery, and trauma are most easily handled just a few feet away in the OB department. Examples are numerous, but the person carrying these babies is unpredictable and at times amusing.

****

The ambulance was bringing in a first time 26-week pregnancy from the adjoining county with sporadic contractions about 2 minutes apart. There was an LPN on board calling in the report. With 20 minutes till arrival time, it included all the keywords for imminent delivery. There was a feeling of tension from both the paramedics and nurse.

The ER prepped for immediate delivery with the option to take the patient to OB if time allowed. Since it was the middle of the night, the OB doctor was called and said he would hurry in from home. The OB department got ready for both regular and C-section delivery. Everyone was tensed and ready for action.

On arrival there was no change in the patient's condition, with contractions still sporadic about 2 minutes apart. The decision was to take her directly to OB. The 20 year-old patient had a tired, haggard look since this had been going on for almost 6 hours, and the last hour consisted of a rough and bouncing ride in the back of the ambulance. The doctor arrived about the same time as the patient and went straight to OB to prep.

Later, the smiling doctor came into ER with the intriguing story that developed in the OB. He said the internal exam had not felt normal, so he had ordered a foley catheter. About 1000cc (a quart) of fluid was drained from her bladder. The contractions stopped and her haggard face turned to sleepy peace. Bladder spasms were causing the feeling of contractions due to twice the amount of an average full bladder. The bladder enlarged to the point of hiding the cervix, causing the "not normal" feeling for the doctor. Further tests found the baby kicking and healthy.

All tensions in the ER were released followed by lots of chuckles and laughter. Many of the same reactions happened in the OB, but out of earshot of the patient. The paramedics and LPN were in route home and also enjoyed the story via radio. The patient left by a side door to avoid embarrassment.

****

A 16 year-old gal came into the ER accompanied by her mother and sister, complaining of lower abdominal pain, vaginal bleeding, and blood clots. Ultrasound indicated a 12-week fetus about to be expelled as a stillbirth. She denied having missed any of her menses saying, "no way can I be pregnant". She was asked if her name was "Mary". She had no idea we were talking of Biblical Times when she denied having that name.

The shocked look on her mother's face was precious but the grin on her sister's face was telltale of knowing more than the mom. The sixteen-year-old "Madonna" was admitted to OB for a D&C while the mother was dealing with the news.

****

The ambulance called in 10 minutes prior to arrival, with a possible miscarriage of pregnancy. In that 10 minutes the miscarriage happened, so the paramedic walked into the ER with a wrapped bundle in a washcloth (not a towel but a washcloth). The

16-week fetus was put into a trauma room with attempts to start the breathing. All failed and he was pronounced a stillbirth.

The mother, looking 10 or 15 years older then her 25 years, was put into another trauma room with preparations to deliver the afterbirth. She announced she was not going to be admitted into the hospital. This was her 4th miscarriage in the past 2 years.

Three hours later she was discharged under Against Medical Advice papers with most of the vaginal bleeding under control. She was a known drug addict but her reason for leaving was she could not miss "work".

The following night she returned on her own, looking like "death warmed over," complaining of weakness even after a short walk. She had spent most of the day in bed unable to get up. Her blood count was low and a blood transfusion was given but she would not stay. She signed out again, AMA. It was anticipated she would return sometime in the near future.

****

A single gal pregnant at 13 weeks said, "I think the baby is in trouble". She said she had felt a lot of pressure "down there" and was now having bleeding along with some contractions. The bleeding was soon classified as "spotting". The ultrasound found the fetus healthy with a beating heart. The diagnosis was "threatened spontaneous abortion". Precautionary instructions were given, like no sex or forceful bowel movements.

The memorable part was the related story of the trip into the ER. Her boyfriend had a suspended driver's license, which necessitated the patient to drive the car. With each "contraction" she would veer all over the road and was eventually stopped by the police. The license on the car was expired, so it was impounded at the scene. The ambulance was summoned to complete the journey. This meant no car.

About 4AM the couple was discharged with no way to get to their home, at least 15 miles away. Three hours later shift change came and went, and they were still in the waiting room. The news related the next evening was that a person came into the ER during the morning shift and heard their story. She offered them a ride home after being seen in the ER.

****

Honeymoon and miscarriage do not go together but that is what happened to a gal from out of town. The good-looking couple came with the bride weeping on the groom's shoulder, while he supported her ambulation. Her wedding had been one week earlier, and a few hours ago she had started having cramps and spotting. She had used a home pregnancy test a week before the wedding, and it did show positive.

An ultrasound test was completed showing she did have a 7-week fetus in the womb, but was not viable. What a way to begin a marriage. She was crying the whole time in the ER with lots of support from her new husband. They were allowed to remain in the room as long as they needed, while waiting for OB to get a bed ready for her.

****

A five-month pregnant 18 year old who had been having pain all day on both sides of her groin stated, "The baby has not been moving for hours". She was worried to the point of tears, which were running down her lily-white cheeks. When asked if she had called her doctor her reply was she did not want to bother him at night. What about during the day? She was too busy.

A special microphone placed on the lower abdomen called a Doppler emitted a loud fetus heartbeat that made everyone smile. Her pain was called "round ligament pain", a normal occurrence of pregnancy. The naive girl who looked more like a child than a late teen said she had never heard that term. The tears dried and were replaced with smiles. The time for teaching was prime.

The nurse took the "significant other's" hand and placed it on the lower abdomen of the mother showing him how the feeling of kicking feet and arm movement can be accomplished. The patient was then shown the same procedures. Both had wide grins and even giggles when they felt the movement. Each additional instruction by both of the nurses was readily absorbed and repeated back with big smiles. It was a happy moment for all.

If the gynecologist personnel did more pregnancy teaching, the ER visits would be greatly reduced. Of course, if that office were asked about each case they would say the teaching had been done.

The couple left happy and thankful.

****

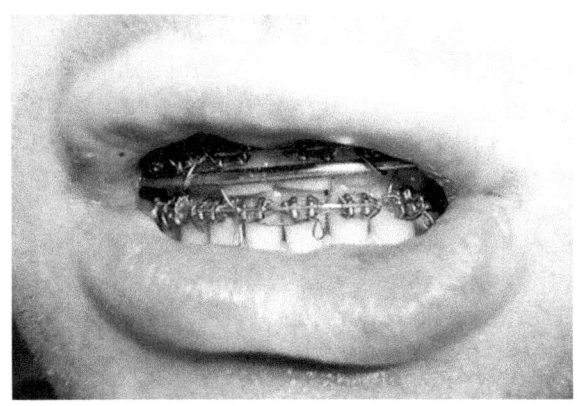

MISCELLANEOUS

What makes a medical patient memorable enough to be placed into a category of 'miscellaneous' and not just listed under a chapter about condition or disease? In this book, the memory would be the same with or without the medical aspect. The addition of a person's condition adds to the memory, but is not a necessity. The 'tough dude crying', the slippery cop-dodging gal, Chester from Gunsmoke, Cupid to a patient's mother, and even the horse-bitten boy episodes could be told in a different setting and still be memorable.

****

He was one tough looking dude, a 38 year-old male, who now was a teary-eyed bundle of self-pity with a high-pitched, whining voice. Two weeks ago he was in a bar- room brawl that caused two teeth to be knocked out, plus a broken jaw. The repair involved his mouth being wired shut and he was put on a liquid-only diet.

He was told the wires could possibly be able to be removed in about ten days. Since he was now on vacation and far from the specialist that who put in the wires, his decision was to remove them himself. He confessed he bought a pair of small wire cutters and started cutting. "I can cut wires as good as some orthodontist", was his excuse. Some of the wire ends were not accessible, so he just left them alone, and went out to have some solid foods.

Soon the chewing action forced the cut ends to embed into the gums, causing extreme pain. His friend said this hulk of a man was actually crying like a baby while in route to the emergency room. He looked like a scolded puppy, with eyes looking upward and his head hanging low. Add tears to that picture and the pathetic scene was complete.

The doctor was able to ferret the embedded wires out of his gums by carefully and slowly pulling and trimming. This corrected the immediate problem of pain. He warned the patient that chewing could easily cause more pain and damage from the remaining wires he had not been able to remove. He must not vary from the liquid diet until cleared by his orthodontist.

The tears had stopped but he still had the puppy-dog look, as he weakly whispered, "No food?"

****

A 35 year-old female came into ER by ambulance from a minor one-car accident complaining of ankle pain. The report from the scene stated no damage to the vehicle and she had a slight limp at the accident scene.

She was sitting upright on the ambulance cot, alert, with a sheepish smile that did not quite fit the situation. She looked comfortable with the halter top and shorter than normal shorts. Her over-abundant makeup was smeared in places but there was no streaking from possible tears. Her breath smelled like she had been at a party, unlike her claim she was going to the party. No matter how minor the accident, she should have been in trouble for drinking and driving.

Pronounced arrogance punctuated each answer to the questions we asked, as her condition was assessed. She admitted having ankle surgery only two weeks ago. Was the complaint of ankle pain from the accident, or the surgery? She huffed and puffed saying she asked for the ambulance just to get away from the accident scene. Why? "Never mind!"

Eventually, she was left alone in the hallway by x-ray waiting her turn. A few minutes later, the technician called ER asking why there was an empty bed sitting there. Around the same time a State trooper came in the main door to get an alcohol test done on her.

She knew she was going to be arrested for DWI and probably taken to jail if a test was done soon, so she slipped out of the hospital without being noticed. By the time they could catch her the blood alcohol had dropped, making the possible DWI charge null and void.

She was found close to the hospital much later, and sure enough the blood test showed only traces of alcohol in her blood. Her ankle was still sore but she refused treatment. The police did not detain her since she did not "break" the law except having the auto accident that caused no property damage. The whole affair was a memorable way to avoid prosecution.

****

It was a holiday weekend and a total of 161 patients had checked into triage the past 24 hours. The average was only 100 patients. Nothing big, bad, or ugly came in, but just lots of patients. The triage nurse who came on duty at 7PM said by 2:30AM she had checked in 67 patients. Due to the long wait, fourteen had left before getting into a room. Some had left after the doctor saw them in a room. They just decided not to wait any longer, and left.

Here was the list of those fourteen patients :

67YO male with 1/4" laceration above his eyebrow.
45YO male who shot a nail gun into his finger.
15YO female with burning urination.
30YO female with a migraine headache for 3 days.
41YO male with a 1/2" laceration on the back of his head.
3 month old that fell off the bed - was playful and cheerful in triage.
30YO female who had a red eye with itch–probably pink eye.
1YO boy with a mosquito bite size puncture wound below the eye caused by a screwdriver. Vision was unhindered.
8YO girl with a small laceration under the chin.
1 month old with tiny cut on the right thumb.
10 month old with cough and "fever" (temp was 98.9)
42YO female with alcohol on her breath who claimed her husband had assaulted her. There was a tiny cut above the right eye. She was begging to have it 'glued' plus some pain

medicine. The doctor said there was not any need to fix it – just let it heal. She went ballistic saying it would cause a scar and then would have to be corrected by a plastic surgeon, and she did not have that kind of money. She was probably 5' 3" and weighed around 180 pounds – she needed to worry about other parts of her body more then her eyelid. When she found out that she was not going to get any narcotic pain pills she grabbed the chart out of the nurse's hand and threw it back, hard! Luckily her alcohol content prevented her from hitting the mark. She stomped out, screaming how lousy it was in ER.

43YO male with chest pain. There was a 3 hour workup on him and when the suggestion was made of being admitted, he refused and left AMA

22YO male with "injured" elbow – no bruise or swelling noted.

It was determined most of the above could easily have waited to see their regular doctor for each problem. The only exception in the list above was the chin laceration of the 8YO girl. A scar is always a concern later in life for a pretty girl.

****

Police "gently" escorted a 35 year-old man into the ER. He was shabbily clothed in a denim shirt and trousers, both stained with brown coffee-like spots mixed with black greasy areas. There was some clothing that appeared wet and smelled like liquor straight from the bottle. His feet were missing shoes, and the socks had holes in the heels and toes. Added to this, his loud, filthy speech made him an unwelcome sight.

When he refused to sit on the edge of the cot, the police shoved a little too hard. That caused the patient to fall backwards off the other side, hitting the floor with a thud. This aggravated him and he began yelling more obscenities and threats of a lawsuit. It was not a pretty scene but he eventually got up and sat on the bed.

The main complaint was neck and head pain that he claimed were caused by the cops. He continued, "They threw me down on the concrete floor and held me there with a knee pushing on the back of my neck. It hurt so bad I must have a big pain shot!" He had been moving his head to extremes like a bobble head doll.

Many warnings were issued telling him if he did not lower his voice and stop the obscenities the doctor would definitely not order a "shot" of any kind. He did lower his voice but the filth kept emitting from those lips when the doctor came into the room.

After a cat scan, which was negative for any injuries, he was offered Tylenol. He said, "Give those to me!" Immediately he aimed and threw them as hard as a drunk can muster toward the nurse, but missed. He then raised his voice again and became even more obnoxious.

Shortly he was being escorted back to jail. The last words he heard from the nurse he tried to hit with the pills was, "Thank you for your visit and don't hurry back."

****

An unassuming 50ish man came to the ER with a right knee twice its normal size. His stiff legged walk brought memories of Chester on the old Gunsmoke TV show. He wore overalls and heavy steel-toed boots with a plaid shirt. He refused a wheelchair saying the pain was worse if he bent the leg.

With a matter-of-fact expression he said in a low voice that the swelling started a few days ago, and now was getting "worrisome". He was guessing all the possible diagnosis' like cancer, arthritis, sprain, and a "dumb accident". As a carpenter, he said it was important in his line of work to have good knees.

An orthopedic doctor was called in which took quite a while since it was late in the night. The patient never complained or even looked anxious during the whole wait. Pain was not in his vocabulary and even a trip to the bathroom did not create a groan or any sign of pain except the slow, stiff legged walk. Numerous offers of coffee, water, and a donut were refused with a calm, "I am fine."

The orthopedic doctor arrived and explained that he was going to stick a big needle into the area around the kneecap to draw off excess fluid. This gentle man replied, "Cool, I want to watch this." When warned it may hurt a lot, he just shrugged his shoulders.

The procedure produced a large amount of thick reddish-yellow fluid and was watched closely by the non-expressive patient. A small frown was noticed once during the most gruesome part.

Most people would be screaming. He admitted the overall pain became less after all the accessible fluid was pulled out. To complete the procedure, he would have to have another procedure to get it all out of the knee.

He asked what caused this condition. The doctor told him it was called "nursemaid knee" named for the women of the past who did the floor scrubbing on their knees. His reply was, "Could we call it "carpenter's knee" instead? It sounds better."

****

A strikingly good-looking single mother brought in her 7 year-old son with a stiff neck. She stated he had fallen out of his top bunk bed the day before and this evening his neck became painful and stiff. Any movement of his head, regardless of direction, was difficult and painful.

Upon returning from getting x-rays the mother asked the nurse about the marital status of that "super cute" technician in x-ray. Not knowing the answer, the technician was requested to go to the room as the mother had a question. This type of request was common but usually it was concerning the x-rays. Not knowing the nature of the request he went without hesitation, asking how he could be of help. The mother became red with embarrassment and uttered something about hurting the nurse who did this. The technician was single and close to her age. It was noticed after a short visit there was an exchange of pieces of paper.

The boy was diagnosed with muscle spasms causing a severe stiff neck. Medications had been given to take the pain away and now were working well. Both mother and son left with a smile.

****

The middle-aged pleasantly plump lady had a sore throat so severe she would "holler", her husband's description, in pain with each cough. Attempts to look into her throat would cause a gag reflex and a heaving session. A strong narcotic pain shot was given that calmed the lady's gyrations, with each breath followed by a shaking spell like a wet dog. Finally a good peek into her throat was successful. There were no signs of redness or even pus pockets so often seen in these types of cases.

A more in depth history was pursued as to when the pain started. Her husband, who had patiently been a quiet observer through all the previous actions and reactions, at this point did all the talking. He said she started complaining yesterday shortly after they finished burning a brush pile. At first he thought it was just normal smoke irritation. The pain kept getting worse during last night and today. She denied any sniffles or coughs the past week.

Her husband then remembered there were some poison ivy plants in the pile and wondered if that may have caused this problem. The doctor had an "ah-ha" moment. He explained the common reaction of poison ivy on the external skin could happen in the throat also. The lady said in a raspy whisper, "If that is it, please do something to make it stop hurting every time I breathe."

Nothing directly could be done to reverse the allergic reaction but the treatments were aimed more at comfort than cure. She readily agreed to be admitted with a poison inhalation diagnosis and lots of medication, just as long as she could breathe easily. In other words, she did not want to "holler" anymore.

****

An elderly man did not tell it like it was and paid the price, but "it all came out right in the end". He said he had pulled into the motel parking lot with a demanding increased urge to "go number 2". The urge had started a few blocks away but now he was desperate to get to the motel room. He got out of the car, and when standing up, got very dizzy. He knew all he had to do was get to the bathroom. He was leaning against the car swaying back and forth hoping for the dizziness to pass.

Seeing his present condition, bystanders insisted he lie down on the ground. He was too embarrassed to say exactly what he needed to do so he complied with their orders. Lying down, the blood returned to his brain and the dizziness lessened. The "urge" was also reduced for the time being.

The ambulance bringing him into the ER reported a possible "AAA" – meaning an abdominal aortic aneurism, a critical situation. The missing sign was a pulsating mass mid abdomen but all other signs and symptoms were consistent with their surmise.

Suddenly, the over-anxious patient was begging for a chance to go to the bathroom and finally confessed his previous urges. He was accommodated with a bedside commode of which he proceeded to forcefully and copiously relieve himself. The smell over-powered the entire ER.

When the gentleman was done the anxious appearance was no longer present in his manner, and he was totally calm. Physically, he was exhausted and only wanted to lie down, which the cat scan allowed. All tests for anything and everything were negative except one. The radiologist reported the scan indicated a completely empty bowel.

Upon discharge he promised never to hold back the full story about anything again, including "number 2". As said in the beginning, "all came out in the end."

****

She was a 15 year-old driver at a go-cart track when her cart came to a stop resulting in a collision from behind, causing "whiplash". According to witnesses, she was in a daze walking out to the parking lot and boarding the waiting church bus. Lying down on a seat, she shortly became unresponsive. There was no change in her condition when the ambulance arrived at the ER. More comments were made of her flaming red hair that fell well below her shoulders then her condition

The first thing done was to try to awaken her using a painful stimulus. It was a knuckle rub on the upper sternum any pseudo unresponsive patient would at least have moved a hand to push away. She did not react. Next her arm was held above her face a few inches and released. Normally a conscious person would instinctively not allow the arm to hit the face but this patient's arm landed right on her nose. A conscious patient faking unresponsiveness would have twitching eyelids – she had no movement of her eyelids.

During the wait of about one hour to complete blood tests with a cat scan, she awoke not remembering anything after the accident. She did recall her go-cart stopping but not the hit from behind. She was so concerned about the loss of recollection she asked over and over, "What happened? Where am I?" She would toss her head around allowing the flaming red hair to float like "red sails in the sunset."

Her pastor was there and explained to her that God purposely made us that way, so the terrible things in life would not vividly haunt us. He added it was a good thing, and to rejoice. A frown appeared on her face at the mention to "rejoice" about being in the ER with a bad headache.

She continued asking for details as to what "really" happened even as she was walking out the door. She would really know what "whiplash" was all about in 24 hours once the severe stiff neck and soreness set in. At least, she would have something to think about besides what "really" happened.

****

About midnight a young gal came limping in with an ankle injury. It looked swollen, but there were a few patients ahead of her. After about a half hour in the waiting room she started to make a fuss about not being seen. She tried to involve the other patients in the waiting room without too much success. She purposely shouted for everyone to hear, "I could drive 40 miles to another hospital, be seen and get home before this dump would do anything."

The triage nurse called that hospital and on the speakerphone had the patient ask the waiting time there. Everyone heard the answer that this type of injury would be approximately an eight-hour wait. This shut her up, and about two hours later she was discharged with an ankle wrap and crutches. No preferential treatment was given her.

The only good bye given her was a sarcastic, "We were happy to be able to have you as a patient, have a great morning." Her reply was only a grunt as the door closed.

****

"What kind of chest pain are you having?" It was the eighth time in the past 6 months this early 30s gal had been into the ER for pain of a migraine headache. In the past she was brushed off and delayed, and in the end not given any of the narcotics that she wanted.

This time there was a new approach. She said the migraine had gotten so bad it was now causing lots of chest pain. She answered our first question with, "It is sharp pain that comes and goes with every heartbeat." "Are you having any nausea or vomiting?" "Yes, I always do with my migraines." "Did you vomit before or after the chest pain started?" "After."

"What is your best guess as to why you are having this chest pain?" "I probably am having a heart attack and if you don't give me some pain medicine I could die." "We only give aspirin for heart attacks." "That won't help me, I have to have something stronger." "Like what?" "Like morphine, or oxycontin, or codeine."

About this time the doctor came in to get an assessment and ordered all the heart attack tests but no medicine. He said it would not be good because we couldn't tell what the pain really was if we killed it with a pill or shot. Her terse and animated reply was, "I have to have a "shot" because that is the only thing that works." "How do you know what works on your heart attack? Have you had heart attacks before?" "No, but I just know."

When all tests came back negative for heart attack and other such symptoms she was offered a Tylenol. As expected, she stormed out of the ER without even signing the discharge papers.

****

Vertigo was the first clinical diagnosis by the nurse for a weak, elderly man complaining of dizziness. . It all had started while he was sitting in the recliner reading a book. He said, "Every time I moved my head the room would spin, and I could not get out of the recliner because it made me so weak."

It was the weakness that became the concern more than the dizziness. "It seems I cannot move, all the energy and strength is gone," was repeated over and over. The medication for vertigo did help the dizziness a small amount, but the weakness continued.

He was a well-dressed man sporting a suit coat and open necked shirt with good conversational skills, who had everyone convinced of the weakness. His skin color was paler then expected and he also pointed out a blue tint in his fingernails. A battery of tests were ordered and his personal physician was called, who happened to be in the hospital making calls. Shortly he arrived and did a thorough assessment, including listening to his heart with a stethoscope.

"Have I ever told you that there was a loud heart

murmur?" asked his doctor. "No, what in the world is that!" replied the patient in a rather scared and uncharacteristic tone. Panic seemed to be setting in on the patient, which was curtailed by the doctor. "It is nothing to worry about, it can be dealt with and you can get your strength back."

The patient did calm down and listened intently to the diagnosis and planned treatments portraying his former stately manner. He was admitted to the hospital with the comment from his doctor, "He is quite a trooper." The patient's reply, "Not when I have these so called 'murmurs' inside of me. Is it like gossiping?"

****

Sharp spurts" was the way a young man explained his stomach pains. Even a drink of special numbing syrup did not change his feeling. He was not fat or skinny, but the way he carried himself made him look a lot older then his 32 years. He looked distraught and depressed but he said nothing about it. One simple question, "Is there anything else bothering you?" broke open the dam of stress and tears.

His wife of 10 years had gone to the store the week after Christmas and never returned. He found out that she ran off with another man and did not take any of her clothes with her, not even one item of her belongings. He had been crying all day and could not sleep at night. No wonder he had gut pain.

He agreed to meet with the psychologist on staff before leaving for home. After some "nerve" medication, he left with his head hanging low and a shuffling walk.

****

A brave and determined looking 12 year-old boy came into the ER with a horse bite on his left shoulder. His denim cowboy shirt was torn, with bloodstains down the sleeved arm. There was a large skin tear and caved in portion of the front part of the shoulder that looked nasty. He said the stallion grabbed his whole shoulder in his mouth, then picked him up and threw him against the stable wall.During the washing and irrigation of the wound, the family was discussing how to tame this horse. The conclusion was to make him a gelding by castration. The boy raised his good arm and said, "I get to do the cutting." Everyone had a good laugh.

****

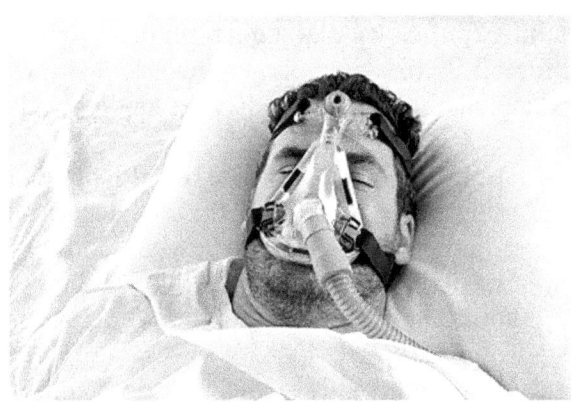

RESPIRATORY

To appreciate "respiratory distress", try breathing a few minutes by pursing your lips around a straw and holding your nose closed. Shortly you will use chest muscles to suck harder on the straw. Following this, you will raise your shoulders toward your ears and puff out your chest to try to make more room for air. The next step is to lean forward and lift up to breathe in, only to hunch over again, on exhalation. Within a short period you get tired of working harder than usual. It is difficult to get enough oxygen to maintain life. Most respiratory patients arrive in the ER because they try to breathe this way for days. They are completely worn out and only want to breathe with ease.

****

A grandmother aged 42 looked much older than her actual years. Her face was crisscrossed with deep furrows; the skin on her face and arms looked like leather with dark blotches; her fingers, ear lobes, and feet were an oxygen starved blue color; her lips were pursed with each exhalation; her eyes were two big statements of anxiety. This was her fourth visit to the ER in the past 6 months. She admitted to two packs of cigarettes per day but her son said it was probably more. This current breathing difficulty had started 3 days ago.

Shortly after arrival to the ER she was on a special machine to do the breathing for her, by placing a tight mask around her mouth and nose and forcefully blowing oxygen inward. Most conversation was with hand signals but some words were understandable through the tight mask.

The first question was why she would do this to herself. "What are you going to do to prevent this?" Her response, "I quit smoking." She pulled up her sleeve to show a nicotine patch. "How long have you been using these?" "3 hours." "When was your last cigarette?" "3 hours ago." "When will be your next cigarette?" "Never."

About 5 hours later with medication both through the mask and by IV she was breathing on her own with reduced effort. She refused to be admitted and was discharged with instructions not to smoke and to see her doctor for frequent check-ups. On her way out the door she was heard telling her son, "I'm having a nicotine fit."

****

She was 70 years old with paper-thin skin coated with cold sweat, making it clammy to the touch. She was breathing about 50 times per minute, creating eyes of despair ready to close for the last time. She was struggling for each of those breaths, which were wearing her down as each minute passed. The ambulance noted the heart monitor was showing pacer spikes meaning she had a pacemaker.

Her oxygen level was near 100% but the problem was the hard work she had to accomplish just to get a breath. She was gasping for each grunt of communication with a repeating, "Help me, Help me". The oxygen mask was not enough, so she was changed to a c-pap machine that forces in the air without the patient having to work for it.

In a few hours she was relaxed, still showing a high percentage of blood oxygen. Her heart was weak, even with the pacemaker. Her diagnosis was congestive heart failure, causing inadequate pumping of blood. She was happy not to have to work for each breath but felt claustrophobic having to wear the airtight mask covering her mouth and nose. Her muffled voice through the mask was understood as, "Thank-you, Thank-you."

She was admitted for further examination to find the reason

why the heart would not pump enough blood, even with a pacemaker.

****

It was an unusually quiet morning in the ER approaching the 5AM hour, when a man's high-pitched voice came from the ambulance bay doors. They had automatically opened for a 45 year-old man on all fours crawling with an arched back, head held high, and pursed lips. In gasping grunts he forced out one-syllable sounds, "as"–"ma"-"t"-"k". When pulled up into a wheelchair he leaned forward so far it started to tip the chair forward into a possible nosedive.

Quickly an aide grabbed his shirt collar pulling back hard, while pushing him into a trauma room. The patient went to his knees beside the cot and laid his upper body onto the bed. A great heave from everyone "flipped" him onto the cot with the backrest in an upright position. As his tee shirt was being cut open, he was given the bare ended oxygen tube turned on at full blast, and told to breathe. His nasal air passage was congested so he shoved the tubing so far into his mouth he gagged, but avoided vomiting. In gasping grunts he indicated a need for a breathing treatment, which was already being prepared.

He got the breathing treatment, plus an IV access to administer more drugs to reverse a severe asthma attack. Shortly a history could be obtained. He lived alone and ran out of his metered dose inhalation medicine the day before, and had been lying in bed hoping for natural relief. He chose to drive himself the 5 miles to the ER with windows wide open to get the cool air of the night, and admitted he had weaved across the whole width of the road many times to get here. When asked if he smoked, the reply was a guilt-ridden whisper, "Two packs a day".

A second breathing treatment was given. By this time he was getting most of his breathing ability back but was so worn out that he fell asleep. About one hour later he was awakened, because his admittance papers were done and he was going to the medical floor. An objection was anticipated but none came.

On his way upstairs he promised never to smoke cigarettes again. Most had heard that before in these situations, but the promise would probably never be fulfilled. Being pushed down the hall to his room he kept repeating, "I promise, I promise".

****

A 59 year-old man had a pronounced "pot belly" and barrel chest reminiscent of an old wood stove. His face, red as a beet, was made worse with each struggling inhalation, and at the same time his shoulders would rise up to the level of his ears. Also, his potbelly would disappear due to the excess abdominal muscle used to take in that precious oxygen.

Shortly techs, nurses and doctors surrounded this man who was about to stop breathing because he had been doing this excess work for 2 days. He was in a critical stage. Blood oxygen level was only 60% before the oxygen mask was strapped onto his face flowing at full blast. IV, blood draws and x-rays were quickly done.

The doctor explained to the patient that he might have to have a tube put into his air passage to help him breathe. A panicky look came over his face and he was able to speak enough to let us know he had been through that before. He pleaded that a c-pap machine be tried first, a tight facemask with pressured airflow through the mouth and nose. His wish was granted, with a warning it might have to change.

The c-pap was set up and shortly his blood oxygen level was 99%. He promptly fell asleep. All staff was also breathing easier as they considered the worst was over. His potbelly remained undisturbed and his shoulders stayed in their proper place.

About half an hour later the blood oxygen level monitor alarm sounded, indicating lower then 90%. Soon it was 85% falling to 78% in a matter of a few minutes. He was awakened and told in no uncertain terms to breathe hard, even with the machine. He was seated in an upright position and shortly placed on the edge of the bed so he could lean forward and be able to raise his shoulders again. Nothing helped an oxygen level of 88 percent was the highest obtained. If his efforts to breathe would slow down, the percent dropped rapidly.

Tears came out of his eyes and ran onto the seal on his face. He knew it was time to be intubated, and this, he did not want. The doctor explained this complication was caused by a "mucus-plug" -

142

nasal secretions that got 'taffy' thick and formed a plug in his windpipe. He reluctantly said yes to the sedation and intubation procedure.

Within the next 3 minutes he was intubated and saline water was put down the tube followed by suction. The first two attempts the suction tube got plugged, but on the third attempt a long, sticky, yellow mucus plug came out, with a truly taffy appearance.

He was admitted to intensive care where more than likely the breathing tube could be removed shortly. He would survive his close brush with death.

****

Do not stand on top of a swivel seat in a boat. That was the lesson a 66 year-old grandfather learned. He and his 8 year-old granddaughter were fishing near shore when her lure got caught on an overhanging limb. The boat was maneuvered under the limb, but standing up in the boat the lure was still out of reach. The 'at-the-moment' solution was to stand on the swivel seat and grab the limb. A small wave rocked the boat, and grandpa came crashing down onto his side on the console. The wind was knocked out of him and his rib pain was excruciating, making it difficult to breathe.

In the ER this lean, muscular former body builder could not breathe without lots of effort. He told the above story adding he was on his knees piloting the boat to the landing some 2 miles away. Most was accomplished by instinct except when he beached the boat at almost full throttle. The sudden stop spilled the granddaughter into the water unhurt. She got onto the shore and ran for help. (No cell phones back then.)

He arrived at the ER by private car driven by a stranger the granddaughter had found. In a raspy whisper he was able to talk in short gasps telling of his pain and difficulty breathing. There were no breath sounds on his right side, indicating a collapsed lung. The chest x-ray confirmed his normally melon size lung had collapsed to the size of a pecan.

The doctor explained his situation and what had to be done to correct it. A large tube would have to be inserted into his side between 2 ribs accessing his chest cavity where the air was under tension. He smiled, saying, "Do anything to help." Shortly he was sedated and the procedure was done. When the hole was made for the tube there was a good "swoosh" of air that rushed out of the chest.

Even though the patient was sedated, his grimacing face disappeared and relief was evident. He would be admitted to the hospital for a few days to allow the lung to re-inflate to melon size.

Later on the ride upstairs his granddaughter was walking beside him, asking if this meant she had lost her fishing lure. With a contagious smile, he said he would be sure to buy her another one.

****

The ambulance report stated a "respiratory distress" case involving a 33 year-old male, soon to arrive. Since that kind of case usually threw up red flags of alert the whole ER crew listened carefully. It was unusual for such a young person to be that seriously in trouble, breathing without trauma. During the transmission of the report the background noise was a constant cough. This was another inconsistency for respiratory distress.

On arrival, the patient was of average height and weight with ruddy facial color and a very tired look. His eyes were drooping, shoulders slumped, arms laid limp along his side, and he had the general look of a wet rag. The cough was non-productive and low in tone. From all indications it was a bad throat irritation or inflammation. Each cough was making the source worse. His blood oxygen level was over 90%, even with all the coughing.

Two breathing treatments followed by a dose of a cough suppressant reduced the cough to about half within the hour. This allowed him to start a long string of repeated "Thank-You's" to anyone that came near. Within another hour the coughing had stopped. He looked relieved and ready for a 'long winter's night of sleep'. Too bad he was admitted, since most of the time sleeping is not an option in a hospital.

****

A 24 year-old Marine and volunteer firefighter saw a neighbor's house on fire. He ran in with a garden hose but could not contain the blaze and had to back out. He inhaled super-heated smoke during the attempt, causing a sore throat, and could only speak in a whisper.

He arrived only able to grunt a few words without coughing and grimacing in pain. His excellent body condition and young lungs free of cigarette smoke were the main reason he was still able to keep going. The top of his head was like a bad hair day due to the excess heat that curled the tips of his hair, even though he had been wearing a cap. His eyebrows were nearly singed away.

Humidified air was administered for a long time to reduce the inflammation in the throat and lung passages. It could take up to 24 hours or more to determine if the damage done to the lungs would cause complications. This meant he had to be admitted. He said he regretted he was not able to save the house. The fire chief reminded him he did the right thing by backing out, saving his own life.

****

It was a busy night when a 60 year-old lady came into the ER with her husband, complaining of shortness of breath and chest pain. Tests were done to rule out congestive heart failure, heart attack and pneumonia. Her heart rate was fast, her breathing was fast, her blood pressure was elevated, and some other signs pointed to a possible blockage of the arteries in her lungs (pulmonary embolus). A cat scan was needed to confirm the diagnosis. She coded on the cat scan table and all efforts to revive her did not work. She died from a blood clot in her lung. The husband went crazy, as could be expected.

The ER doctor was looking at all the nurse's notes, the lab reports, and x-rays to try to determine where he may have missed something. It was a 'walking on egg shells' time for all the staff when it came to dealing with him.

One half hour later it was his turn to take the next new patient when a 38 year–old lady came into the ER hyperventilating and complaining of chest pain. Her heart rate was fast, her breathing was fast, and her blood pressure was elevated. The doctor took one look at her anxious face and ordered a blood thinner and high flow oxygen before any extra tests were completed. He made the right call and the patient was diagnosed with a blood clot in her lung and eventually made a full recovery.

So which one was more memorable? It probably was the

combination of one reinforcing the other that was etched in the memory of each staff member, including the doctor.

****

A "prim and proper" lady with a great attitude slowly walked into the ER complaining of a "slight" shortness of breath. From the outset she was apologizing for any trouble, but it was out of "concern" for her friends tagging along behind her slow walk.

She had bypass heart surgery a few weeks prior, and overall was feeling better than before. She was not overweight for her nearly six-foot height and 60 years. A small amount of make-up accented her high cheekbones, long eyelashes, and smiling lips.

The heart sounds on her left side were muffled and her breath sounds on that side were faint. A chest x-ray confirmed suspicions of a pericardial effusion (fluid accumulation around the heart), which was not uncommon after heart surgery. The correction was for the cardiologist to insert a needle into that area and pull the fluid out. It was going to be a long wait to get the doctor to the ER because he was in surgery at the time.

This quiet and unassuming lady just waved her hand in a relaxed motion saying that she did not have anything else to do and could wait. Her friends had a different idea about the long wait. Her reply to them indicated she was in charge of her wishes, as she asked them to wait in the waiting room. This allowed most of the crew to interact with her and get to know her better. Most of her requests and desires were gladly granted just because she was so nice and compliant. Any requests not able to be done were answered with a wave of the hand saying, "Perfectly fine." Oxygen did the most for her comfort and she took a nap.

About 3 hours later the cardiologist got out of surgery and came to do the pericardiocentesis. She had instant relief from her breathing difficulties, and with large theatrical movements the doctor removed her nasal cannula for the oxygen. The "ear to ear" smile on her face gave everyone a good feeling and sense of a job well done. She thanked everyone and walked briskly out of the ER to join her friends to go home.

****

The sounds of stridor belonged to a 16 year-old gal accompanied by her mother, as they moved along the corridor to the ER. This is a high-pitched sound that grows louder with each inhalation, more common for a young child than a teenager. It is a respiratory emergency and has to be treated carefully. In this case the patient was carefree, and with a smile, would produce this new high-pitched sound in different ways to entertain herself and upset her mother. She whispered, "But it doesn't hurt."

The ER doc told her to stop upsetting her mother because this condition could cause a gagging spasm in the throat and prevent her from breathing altogether. He took a quick peek into her throat, but was careful not to aggravate a gag reflex and cause that dreaded spasm. He called in the ENT doctor.

After an hour of constantly reminding the pretty blond not to make more noise then necessary, the doctor arrived. He had called in orders for a special breathing treatment and an IV to administer anti-inflammation medicine. The high-pitched sound had improved to a mid range tone and there was only slight inflammation on examination by the ENT. After six hours of constant breathing treatments and medications her near normal breathing and voice had returned, allowing her to go home.

16 hours later the same girl and her mother came back into the ER with a much different worried demeanor. The high-pitched "Johnny-one-note, EEEEEEeeeeeee" of her voice was a higher pitch then the previous night, plus she could not whisper.

The ENT again found little inflammation in her throat and realized it may be connected to stress, more this time then the day before. She acknowledged by a nod of the head she was scared, and afraid she might die because of what she had been told the last time. She also had a history of panic attacks.

A nerve medication was given IV since she could not swallow a pill. In about a half hour she was relaxed, and her inhalation pitch was much lower with a good whisper.

She still had some inflammation and was told to continue that medicine and take the nerve pill when she felt uptight, or the stridor started.

The improvement of her physical condition also improved her demeanor, so she was back to playfully teasing mom again. With a side-glance at her mother she would produce a small high-pitched sound. Mother would jerk her head in a startled fashion, immediately followed by a giggle from the patient.

****

"Don't ruin my chances in the Mr. Universe contest," uttered the 89 year-old patient. He had just been informed that a hole would be made in his side between the ribs, and a hose placed inside his chest. His expression did not change for a minute, then a big grin appeared as he glanced back and forth between everyone present.

The ambulance had found him at home on the bed with blue colored lips and fingernails, gasping for each breath. Tests did show pneumonia on the right side and a partially collapsed lung on the left. He needed a chest tube to allow the lung to re-inflate.

His history indicated he had been an emphysema patient for 20 years with many ER visits over the years. "I kind of like it here when I am in trouble, but to poke holes in my side is not something I care for." Tears appeared in the corners of his big brown eyes as he went on, "Does this mean I am going to die soon?"

"Not if I can help it." the doctor replied. "Good, just get me to my next birthday, stated the patient. I want it to be known that I lived to 90." "When is your birthday?" With a smile, he said, "Tomorrow." "We can do that," said the doc.

The last update report from the floor was 2 days later and he was still going strong, saying, "Mr. Universe, here I come."

****

A 53 year-old lady arrived in triage by herself, stating, "I am having a tough time breathing." She was not struggling or having any other signs of respiratory distress. She had a bright congenial smile, and her eyes sparkled as she looked around.
It appeared she was dressed to go out on the town, complete with a long dress, heels, and dark hair draping across the shoulders of her silk blouse.

Her history was unimpressive, except for the past few weeks she had some periods of "slight" breathing problems lasting less than a day. This time it continued more than a day, and according to her was "more pronounced". Her pulse was slightly elevated and her blood oxygen saturation was in the low 90s. The situation did not seem an immediate emergency and she was put into the waiting room to await her turn.

After a short time she was seen getting up from her chair and slowly making her way back to the triage nurse, while hanging onto the back of each chair in the row for support. Her smile was now a frown, her eyes were shouting "pending doom" and a pale skin color was prominent. A single utterance in a whisper, "Help", created a flurry of action.

Quickly a wheelchair was provided, as she indicated she thought she was going to pass out. Shortly a room was made available and oxygen was applied, while she sat, leaning forward on the edge of the cot. Her saturation was now 86%.

The oxygen mask was causing a suffocating feeling but shortly she started to feel better, and with encouragement decided to tolerate that feeling. In a few minutes her breathing rate slowed to half and the color returned to her skin. A little spark flickered in each eye as the saturation climbed to 98%.

Her gratitude for the quick lifesaving efforts not only were expressed at the time, but many times over the next few days in the hospital while she recovered from congestive heart failure, anemia, (low red blood cells), and thrombocytopenia.

When she visited the ER after discharge from the hospital, she was once again the beautiful, bright-eyed lady with a congenial smile who came into the triage area just a few days earlier. She was in her long dress, silk blouse, and heels. She thanked everyone for saving her life because she thought for sure she was going to die.

Looking down at her dress and shoes she added, "As long as I am dressed for the evening I might as well go out and celebrate. Anyone want to join me?" Sincere apologies were the only answer she got in return, since the shift was only beginning.

****

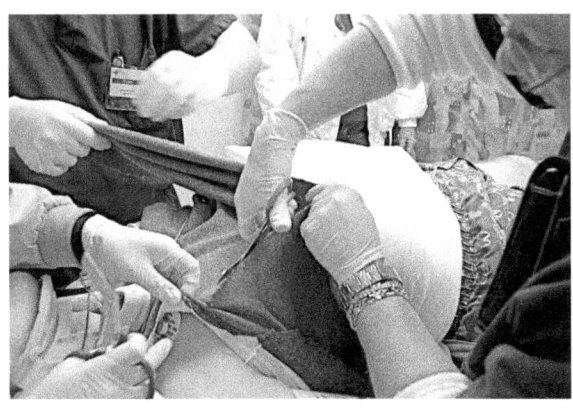

<u>TRAUMA</u>

People think most of the activity in the ER consists of gunshots, major auto accidents, and other life or death incidents commonly called Trauma. Small hospitals have a low percentage of their total patients seen as "true" trauma cases. All major cases are memorable, but what makes some more so than others? The actions and reactions of the patient to the situation make the difference. Since it is a once in a lifetime experience for most patients, there is no past reference to know how they are expected to react. Some think they are dying and resolve to quietly go. Others may fight as never before to remain alive. Possible loss of limb, sight, or function brings different attitudes and reactions. The extremes of these reactions are what makes the patient memorable.

****

A new $17,000 Harley-Davidson motorcycle was an awesome sight until it went out of control on a curve as a result of loose gravel under the tires. The mid-30s man with his wife aboard went into a deep ditch, running head on into a culvert. The epitome of all motorcycles was damaged beyond repair. The owner was seriously injured including a short period of unconsciousness. His wife was seriously injured, but to a lesser degree.

He arrived by ambulance with his large-framed, muscular body covered with mixed dried and fresh blood. The blood made his face resemble a gruesome mask. He realized he was seriously injured but was amazingly calm while strapped tight to a backboard, with a cervical collar to prevent any head movement. The matter-of-fact tone of constant questions of concern for his wife got vague answers since they were unknown at the moment. He thought she was alive, but the way his questions were asked it was obvious he feared the worst.

The pain tolerance level must have been extremely high for this big man since there were cuts and scrapes from chin to forehead, leaving his nose hanging by a thin strip of skin. There was a large laceration on the back of his head, and swelling on the side of the head. His right foot angled off to the side, due to multiple fractures of both lower leg bones. A narcotic pain med was given by IV, but for most people the whole cabinet of meds would not be enough.

X-rays and cat scans confirmed most of the suspected fractures of the cheekbones and legs, plus 3 broken ribs. His helmet had come off after the initial impact with the culvert but had probably prevented brain damage, looking at the gouges and scrapes on its' surface. The only comment the tolerant patient could make was, "This is what I get for riding after drinking."

Later, his wife was able to come into the room in a wheelchair to visit, after completing her minor treatments. Once he knew his wife was ok, his tolerance to pain suddenly disappeared and he was begging for more pain medication of any kind.

He was quiet, obedient, and willing to do anything asked during his four-hour stay in the ER. He was then admitted to the surgical floor for orthopedic procedures and eventual plastic surgery on his face. It was a perfect trauma case for any "adrenaline-rush-seeking" nurse, especially since the patient was most cooperative.

****

Late at night in the dorm room after a long study session for finals, the roommates decided to let off some tension. A friendly wrestling match resulted in one student's foot being severely twisted, producing a loud "snap" and then a crunching sound. During the ambulance ride, the patient was documented as "crying like an ape with a bullhorn."

The EMTs slowly wheeled the patient into the ER, trying not to jar or bump the cot, as that would produce another loud bellow from the depths. There was no doubt in anyone's mind the protruding bone thru the skin immediately above the ankle spelled compound fracture. The bleeding was controlled, but the student was not concerned with such things just then.

The sedative and other medications were in full force ,allowing this once suffering person to become a slobbering, slurred-speech kid. It was time to pull, twist, and maneuver the wayward foot back into place. The once jabbering person became a screaming and hollering mess again. The protruding bone disappeared inside the large laceration, and the foot was back in the upright position ready for a temporary splint.

Memory is a funny thing in these cases. About 10 minutes later the patient "awoke" with no recollection of the screams and hollering during the reduction of the fracture. He insisted, "Nothing in this world would make me say the things my roommate said he heard." His roommate had been waiting in the hallway. He was willing to make outrageous bets concerning the matter.

He was admitted for surgery, which would include metal plates and screws.

****

In the wee hours of the morning an 18 year-old young man walked into the ER holding a bag of frozen peas to his chin. (His mother had been told that peas were better then a bag of ice.) The injury was caused by an auto/tree collision at 3 in the morning. A lower tooth was shoved completely through the lower lip leaving a ½ inch horizontal laceration on the outside.

After she was told her son would be ok, the worried mother asked, 'Will this injury affect the playing of his horn?" She added, "He placed high in previous contests, plus he is in the upper 10% of his graduating class. He does not drink, smoke, or do illegal drugs and is a straight "A" student." She did make her point as to the character of her only boy. She told us he was going to compete in a statewide competition.

Further examination of the lower lip found a large tear along the inner lip and gum juncture. The patient could push his tongue over his lower teeth and inside the lower lip quite easily, theoretically down to the inside of his chin area. This meant he would not be able to play his instrument until this tear healed completely – about 3 or 4 weeks. Any forceful blowing or even laughter could possibly re-tear the injury. In other words, there would be no competition participation next week.

The mother was devastated when she was told the situation. When the boy was told, he remained stoic and later privately confessed, "I really didn't want to go to that boring concert thing anyway." However, he maintained a good acting performance for the benefit of his mother concerning his "disappointment".

Stitches both inside and outside the lower lip were completed and he was discharged. After they left ,the question remained: what was an honor student with no blemishes of character doing out at 3AM on a weekday of school? The answer will be known to only he and his parents, as it was ethically not asked or volunteered in ER.

****

Adrenaline-induced images popped into everyone's mind as the ambulance report started out that the 40 year-old patient was "gorged by a bull." This called for a demonstration of what "ER" was all about. The radio transmission had no background noise except the siren wailing and the road noises of the fast- moving ambulance. He must be unconscious. The verbal report continued, "The patient is conscious and alert with bleeding controlled." How could that be?

The patient arrived lying on his side, talking like nothing had happened. He had to finish his story to the paramedic about how awesome the horse was that he bought this past week. Then the patient gave permission for the staff to hear the full report of his injury.

He was a tall, chunky man in a cowboy shirt and what remained of his denim jeans after being cut from belt loop to hem on the right leg. The left leg of his jeans was still intact with a cowboy boot still on his foot. He was calm with a "matter of fact" attitude, while saying that he just needed to be stitched up and he would be on his way.

He was one tough dude. The horn of the bull caught his upper thigh, ripping flesh about one inch deep into the hamstring muscles, and extending about 6 inches up into his buttocks. It lay open about one inch wide exposing tendons, nerves, and blood vessels. Every time he tried to move his lower leg the action of the muscles and tendons was readily apparent, giving all a good lesson in upper leg anatomy. He said he flew through the air "with the greatest of ease" landing on his right shoulder, which was a "tiny bit sore". Being the aforementioned "tough dude" his "tiny bit sore" was taken as a possible broken shoulder.

X-rays showed no broken bones or dislocations even in the right shoulder. A surgeon admitted him directly to the OR for irrigation and repair of the wound.

A final comment he made was in defense of the bull, "When the attack occurred, I was leading him to the barn for castration."

****

Weird, unusual, freaky, and amazing are just a few of the terms that might have described the case of the drilled breast. It happened late one night as a 30 year-old woman was helping her husband put tools away. She was loosening the chuck of a drill with the chuck wrench, the curved rod that has the gears on one end. The trigger was touched as she held the drill directly in front of her. The drill did a quick spin throwing the chuck key off and drilling directly into her right breast. It was spinning when it tore thru her sweatshirt and bra, causing fabric to be carried into the flesh along with the steel rod.

She slowly and carefully walked into the ER with both hands carefully cupping the breast to lessen the pain. She looked scared, with eyes huge in her face and a mouth that held a firm "O" shape. It had been a long drive for her husband trying to avoid any bumps and taking curves slowly. She said her arms were aching trying to hold everything still to minimize any further damage. She was 26 weeks pregnant and had a great fear of not being able to breastfeed on the right side since the entry point was about 1 inch above the nipple.

When she was wheeled to an exam room and laid down, the only person available to relieve her aching arms and hands was the male nurse assigned to the room. He carefully replaced her cupping hands with his own and held very still. Her husband remained calm, wearing a wide grin and eyeballing the nurse.

It took about a half hour to assemble all the anticipated equipment needed to be ready for the removal of the object. The worst fear was a possible arterial bleed. During that time the nurse and patient talked about all kinds of subjects, trying to avoid the implications and suggestions the situation could conjure. Once, and only once, her husband asked if she was enjoying all this intimate attention. The glare thrown his direction had an emphatic "be quiet" tone.

The doctor was ready and the nurse opened his cupped hands just enough to allow removal of the chuck key. All the tension and anticipation turned into a huge disappointment. Because the curved key was spinning when it entered the skin, it did not go deep but had tunneled just under the skin. There were just a few drops of blood and only one suture needed to close the hole. She would definitely have a large bruise at the site but nothing else. She was also assured breastfeeding would be part of her new baby's life.

Now it was the patient's turn to make comments about how the nurse was going to explain his night's experiences in the ER to his wife. She did leave for home in much the same position as when she arrived – cupping the sore breast in both hands.

****

"Two in one shot" was how the husband and wife described the gunshot accident injuring her left hand and his right hand. Her ring finger was dangling from the base with a deformed wedding ring filling the void. His injury was in the pad area at the base of his right thumb. Both had bleeding under control.

She was 40 years old with extra weight here and there that added to her beauty more than taking away. Her fingers were short and chubby making the wound appear less then it really might be. The tears of pain were rolling off her high cheekbones as she begged for some pain relief. Instead of the expected hysterical cries for help we heard a deep throated gurgling resulting from holding back the screams with contorting facial grimaces. She cradled her hand in the crook of her right arm as the doctor injected numbing solution near the wound. Pain relief was shortly achieved.

Her story of the events matched that of her husband who was being assessed in another room. She had been looking at a revolver when it slipped out of her hand. Both she and her husband grabbed for the gun, causing it to fire. It was believed the bullet passed thru her finger and into his hand. An x-ray and probe could not find a hole in his hand and there was no exit wound. Our second guess was the hammer on the gun could have caused the supposed gunshot wound.

The husband was discharged with 2 stitches and a big bruise. His wife had a compound fracture of the ring finger and lots of nerve, tendon and vessel damage. Her pain was under control and she was admitted for surgical repair. Her new concern was how she could ever wear the wedding rings again, no matter how good the doctor was with the stitches. She was calm compared to the expected reactions seen in similar painful cases, which made it a delight to help her.

****

Words like young, immature, overweight, arrogant, demanding, and just a misguided kid were some of the thoughts that came to mind. He was only 20 years old, but stupid would be the best word to look up in the dictionary to find his true name. He had been arguing with his brother at 2 AM when he lost his temper. He kicked the patio door, shattering the glass. As his foot passed through the broken glass it caused a large laceration near the ankle. Bleeding was not severe since the artery was missed, but a tendon was severed, as clearly seen inside the wound.

During the examination it was noticed he could move his foot a little in the direction that tendon would control. A closer look inside the wound showed the severed ends of the tendon were about ½ inch apart with a piece of fatty tissue adhered to each end, much like a noodle would hold a broken rope in place.

When "stupid" was told he had to be admitted to repair the tendon, he denied the need since he could move the foot in all directions. He was advised he could go home but only after he walked across the room. He jumped off the bed onto the floor causing the piece of fatty tissue to release the foot, making it flop around without a purpose. Screams followed, and a sudden leap back onto the bed made a thud, landing with his foot flying out of control. He was now a believer of the doctor's words   In fact, he was almost in shock from then until he went to the operating room.

****

"I've been shot – real bad!!!" The hysterical 26 year-old man cried as he came through the ambulance doors of the ER.

This was preceded by a horn -blowing pickup that drove into the bay, sounding like a large flock of flying geese. He was holding his right side and bending forward with a ghostly pale look on his face as he walked in, real slow. His repeated in a high-pitched voice, "I've been shot, I've been shot!"

The first priority was to find the entrance and exit wounds which were on the right side of the abdomen and right side of the back respectively. The repeating phrase was then replaced by a low, scared voice, "Am I going to die? Am I going to die?" When the firm and convincing 'no' answer finally took hold the patient calmed to a shaking and crying mass of jello. Every action and reaction he displayed was based on fear.

After all the gunshot protocol procedures were done he was given a sedative and allowed to sleep until the surgeon arrived. It still was not known if any vital organs were involved, and an exploratory surgery was needed in the operating room. His vital signs remained stable.

A report later said only fatty tissue outside the vital organ area was involved, and the patient was all smiles flirting with every nurse that came into his room. The ER did not learn the details of how and why in regards to the shooting.

****

At 1 AM, the ambulance arrived with a 16 year-old girl involved in a car rollover down a steep embankment. She was on her way home from a night job when she fell asleep at the wheel. A passer-by saw the headlights shining upward from below and made a phone call to 911. First responders quickly arrived on the scene and stabilized the girl. EMS strapped her to a backboard with a cervical collar in place.

She arrived in the ER with an entourage of calm adults following. They were the three first responders and had a special concern in this case. They were the patient's grandfather, and her mother and father.

After an hour of x-rays the diagnosis was no injuries – not even a scratch. She was told it must have been the special care she got from her rescuers that led to the great outcome. She agreed with a big grin, and her family was saying a lot of "Whews".

The 90 year-old patient of a nursing home was transferred to the ER by ambulance with a complaint of left hip pain. The nursing home report stated she had not fallen but could not bear any weight on her left leg. The lady had some dementia problems and insisted she had not fallen

She was a lovingly sweet person with a big smile during the times she was not moving or being moved. She did not scream but would make terrible life- threatening expressions when she was transferred first from the ambulance cot to the ER bed, then to the x-ray table and back. Her skin was paper-thin showing a 10-inch long bruise along the left thigh that looked more than a few hours old. She still did not confess falling when asked about the bruise.

Her femur was broken in the main shaft area in three places with fragments scattered throughout the fracture area. In other words, it was a major blow or fall that caused this much damage. It would be major surgery to fix it ,if that was possible at her age.

She was packaged up in a special traction splint for transfer to another facility. When the patient was told she was being sent to see a geriatric orthopedic surgeon, she wanted to know what that meant. When told it was a bone doctor for "old" people, she replied, " I am NOT OLD!" followed by one of her big smiles. Shortly, it was replaced by that life-threatening expression when she was moved to the ambulance cot.

Late one evening a tour bus pulled up in the ER parking lot to deliver an injured passenger. The 77-year-old lady was embarrassed to be brought to the ER this way, but she was assured it was normal. She had a makeshift sling on her left arm with the blouse unbuttoned enough to take her left sleeve off. Her first comment was, "Please, don't cut my good blouse".

She was a spry, chipper lady who talked long sentences in one breath. In about one minute she explained the whole accident in detail using only one breath. She slipped on a stair landing on the parking lot, left elbow first. She said, "Pain is doing me in but I can take it if I have to."

The deformed look of her upper arm was not a displaced

humerus, but a large hematoma - blood clot. There was a simple fracture just above the elbow with some chip fractures of the elbow. The bruise was starting to get distinct in the elbow area.

Her jaws would clamp tight and her eyes would close whenever she had to move or be moved. More and more narcotics were given until she felt "comfortable". Finally, a fiberglass splint was in place with a professional sling to support it. There was no emergency to get it repaired, so treatment could wait till she got home on the bus tour leaving the next day. She was told to take care, and she said, "With all those old people on the bus I will be 'mothered' and taken care of like no one could imagine."

****

She was only 7 years old, but a true heroine. A pick-up started to roll downhill with her 4 year-old brother near an open door on the truck. She grabbed him and pushed him out of the way, but slipped on the gravel and landed in the path of the front tire. Her upper legs were run over after being pushed along the rocks a short distance.

She arrived at the ER on her mother's lap in the seat of that same pick-up, as her father carefully took her in his arms for a transfer to an ER wheelchair. A large towel was draped across her upper legs. She stopped her crying and occasional scream only to plead, "I don't want to see it". Quickly she was put in a trauma room with two doctors and auxiliary personnel.

She continued crying while her parents tried to comfort her. The towels were removed after a sheet was draped across her waist area to prevent her being able to watch. Both upper legs looked like hamburger with ground in dirt and pebbles. Each had a large laceration in the midst with bleeding under control. Her left hand was scratched with a deformed little finger, the only bone fracture.

She understood most everything she was told that had to be done. Her only reply was, "OK, just don't hurt me any more." When her parents asked her if it was ok to leave while personnel cleaned her sores she replied, "I want you to stay, but I don't want you to hear me cry - so leave." That indicated to everybody she was mature for her age.

Conscious sedation was given allowing her to endure the procedures. The sedation did not take away pain so she reacted to the cleaning of the wounds almost as she had without sedation, but luckily, she would not remember anything. The surgeon had determined it was not serious enough to take her to the operating room.

The patients from the front of the ER to the back could easily hear her pleads and screams. One lady said tears were streaming down her own cheeks in sympathy. Narcotic pain medications were also given to lessen the pain but with a child it was a delicate balance.

When the cleaning was done and the numbing medicine in the lacerations were doing their job, this made the suturing possible without a sound since she fell asleep for the last hour of the three hours she was being repaired. Her parents were allowed in and shortly after the stitches were completed her sedation wore off. She became fully awake with lots of questions. "What happened?" "Is it fixed?" "Did I cry?" "Did I scream?" "What are they doing now?" "Can I go home now?" There was not a doubt the sedation had worked just as it was supposed to work.

Later, it was discovered there were two simple fractures of the pelvis that would keep her off her feet for two weeks or more. She was transferred to a pediatric specialist in a town 3 hours away. Her questions of "what", "when", "how", and "why" were still coming one after the other as she left for the long trip.

****

"It hurts so much, I can't move my arm", was the repeated complaint of a middle-aged lady being wheeled into the ER. The paramedics said she was saying the same thing over and over all the way in the ambulance. The report from the scene told of a broadsided accident into the passenger door where the patient was riding. After a good dose of pain medication and x-rays, she felt better. Diagnosis was a crushed right elbow and a broken radius bone.

Her pain still at a high level, this attractive 48 year-old lady was now only making that same statement every minute, instead of constantly. She also added, "Why does it hurt so much?" The doctor took her good elbow and pressed on the end saying, "Notice how rounded and hard this bone feels?" He then instructed her to reach across her body with the left arm and touch the same place on the bad elbow. "It feels like a marshmallow." She then knew how much damage had been done.

The surgeon looked at the x-ray, shook his head, and told the patient he would fix it, but did not know for sure how until he got in there to get a better look. Her only concern was, "Will it still hurt?" The dreaded answer was, "Yes, for a while." Her predictable reply was, "Oh, well."

It was reported the following day the surgery took nearly 5 hours. Results were not known, as it was in so many cases in the ER.

****

Doing the splits was not on the 39 year-old pleasantly plump woman's agenda. She accidentally did the gymnastic maneuver when her right foot caught in the last stair step and her left leg went out in front of her. She said she heard a loud "pop" as her buttocks hit the ground. The loud crying was for the pain, but, as she put it, "I can't walk, I can't put my legs together, it hurts." Each leg was draped off opposite sides of the ambulance cot.

There was a large bulge half way down the back of her left upper leg that was soft and tender. The worst pain was higher up near the buttocks. A bone fracture was ruled out, leaving a diagnosis of torn hamstring muscles. The soft bulge was internal bleeding, causing a hematoma (blood pool) below the tear.

She kept repeating she could not walk, even after 2 hours of x-rays and exams. She was told there were no injuries preventing her from standing on at least one leg. "But I can't, there is no way." Long reasoning discussions finally paid off and she sat on the edge of the bed with the back of both legs pressed against the mattress. That position was only momentary, with a loud, "Oh, my God that hurts so bad" followed by a leap upward to take the pressure off the hematoma. The result was a woman in upright standing position.

"Hey, it feels better this way." She would not sit down or lie down the rest of the time it took to discharge her. She even walked out to the car using the crutches provided, with a huge ice pack ace bandage wrapped onto the back of her left leg. Getting into the car was a series of "OOoo", "Aahh", and a few screams as she carefully slid into the back seat lying on her right side and holding her left leg up on the back of the back seat. Her friend commented on the "unlady-like position" which got a quick quip, "Shut up and drive!"

****

It was a few hours after midnight. The police scanner began broadcasting a brawl in progress in a residential neighborhood. It was normally a clue that the ER was going to get 2 patients that had to be kept far apart during their visit.

Two ambulances arrived about 5 minutes apart. One held a raggedly dressed middle-aged man, obviously drunk, and the other held an older, well dressed man who was joking about how he got the best of his opponent. The ER was near empty and the separation was far enough apart so that the homeless drunk did not hear the bragging of the "winner". The doors to each room were closed, just to be sure the words did not carry to the inebriated man's ears that might aggravate a clearly deranged mind.

"I clobbered him good with that dang pipe he used on me," was the older man's abbreviated description of the events. "He swung only once and with my 'fast reflexes' I grabbed the pipe just as it bounced off my chest." The same time he was talking, his wife was nearly screaming, thinking her husband was going to die because that stupid man had hit his pacemaker.

The 58 year-old patient laughed and said he felt just fine. The mark on his left upper chest was just an inch away from his pacemaker site. The paramedic said they did not see any pacer indication on their heart monitor, but his pulse was a weak 90 beats per minute - a little high. Neither he nor his wife knew what the pacemaker was set. The full EKG reading did show pacer marks at the 90 beats per minute rate.

The patient finally quit bragging long enough to tell the story of how the fight came about. Walking home from his job as a night auditor in a motel, he saw a man urinating on the front door of a neighbor's home. When he confronted the man in the dark he did not notice the man's free hand held a two-foot length of pipe. "In one move he swung the pipe around and hit me, but I was good and caught it in mid air. Then I swung at him with the dang pipe, but missed. My fist did not miss, as I got him in the stomach he went down. I was screaming for my wife at the same time. We scuffled on the ground until the cops came," he concluded, with his nose high in the air showing pride.

All tests came back negative and since the patient was not having any symptoms of a fast heart rate he was discharged and was still bragging of his prowess as a "protector of the neighborhood". His opponent was taken to jail.

****

A waitress at a local restaurant came in with tears in her eyes, a grimace on her face, but a smile on her lips. It was an unusual combination, but the story was even more unusual. Her hand was wrapped in a white cloth napkin showing a large area of red bloodstain.

She had been at the salad bar putting ice under the salad pan while holding it up with her left hand high enough for the scoop to fit under. It slipped, landing on her right hand. The stainless steel pan had a rather sharp edge that did all the damage as it landed.

"It was so stupid", she told the doctor as calmly as possible. "The only thing I could think of saying to the people in the salad bar line was to watch out for blood in your salad . Sounds kind of dumb now."

She would not let anyone unwrap the napkin, afraid of the pain it might cause. She slowly and carefully unwound the cloth, exposing the ice cubes contained inside. "Wow, it is worse than I thought. When it happened, I just grabbed some ice and the napkin and got here as quick as possible. I wouldn't even let my boss see it. I just told him it was bad. And it is bad."

The little finger was hanging off to the side with a near amputation wound just above the first knuckle. There was a deep wound on the ring finger also. Blood started to ooze out again.

The surgeon determined a tendon had been severed and the whole finger needed to be repaired in the OR. It was going to be a difficult recovery for a right-handed gal. She was a single mother with 2 children and having to miss one day of work would be bad, not to mention several days. Her bigger concern at the moment was whether she would lose her job.

****

At 79 years, she admitted being an "Okie" from Tulsa all her life,. She was holding her left arm tight against her body with her right hand cupping her elbow. Her son, who brought her into the ER, said she never complained, but tonight she kept saying, "It hurts".

Earlier when stepping out of his pickup, she either tripped or slipped making a two point landing, left hip and left shoulder. She said, "My hip is just fine, oh, maybe a little sore, but my shoulder doesn't feel so good. It was such a stupid accident. It's going to ruin my visit with my son and his wife."

It was obvious x-rays were going to be needed so the undressing started. The nurse tried to replace the right hand with his by holding onto the mid upper arm. The "yelp" had a piercing tone but it was not a scream. The upper arm bone just flopped around with bone ends grinding together making a terrible sound called "crepitus". Any normal person would have been screaming but she was tolerating horrible pain.

When she was told the clothes would have to be cut off she insisted it would be ok to take off her blouse. After a few more tries she quietly agreed cutting might be better. She was permitted to keep holding the elbow during the whole procedure, per her request.

When she came back from x-ray her only comment was, "They are not so nice down there - they made me remove my hand and it really hurt." The fractured upper arm was in 3 pieces that needed surgery. The reaction to that diagnosis was as calm and reserved as all her other actions. Some people have high tolerance to pain and then some add perseverance of attitude to that. She was admired for her toughness but she had been sweet at the same time.

****

According to the State Troopers, the 40 year-old lady's story of her injuries did not make sense. Her right wrist was hurting and there were road scrapes on the side of her face. She insisted she tripped and fell while walking. The evidence said something else.

"I was riding with my boyfriend and his kids in the car. We were arguing and I didn't want to be yelling at him in front of his children." She indicated this scenario had also happened in the past. "So I got out of the car to walk it off. In a few minutes he would normally let me back in the car, but this time he drove off." The location she indicated was not where they found her.

They found her tennis shoe 10 feet away from where she had

been found. Her excuse was, "When I tripped, my shoe must have come off." They found her 2 miles from where she said it happened. Again she reasoned, "I must have walked farther then I thought." The boyfriend never showed up at the ER or even called. "He had the kids, and had to stay with them."

X-rays and exams indicated no injuries. The scrapes on her face were treated and a wrist brace was applied.

The trooper surmised the boyfriend pushed her out of the car while still moving and then drove off. She denied nothing like that happened, as so many gals will do when abused. It would be interesting to know what really happened but nobody will ever know.

****

It was 3 AM when the ambulance doors opened, allowing a robot-like patient to enter, holding his head in both hands. Tears were streaming down both cheeks from reddened eyes and he had a worried expression. There was a streak of blood down his forehead, dripping off his nose onto the floor. There was no sideways or up and down movement with each step.   His footsteps were like someone trying not to break eggshells on the floor. This was an unusual concept for a 17 year-old kid, obviously in good physical condition ,dressed only in swimwear.

His head and neck were quickly stabilized with a special collar before the whole story was told. His girlfriend said, "It started with some pills and liquor that made him extra daring without any thought of the consequences. He thought he was at the deep end of the swimming pool and dove into the water. It was the 3 foot end and I guess he hit his head on the bottom."

There was a laceration on the top of his head starting at the hairline and extending about 3 inches back. Bleeding was somewhat controlled. He proclaimed, "My neck hurts real bad. Did I break my neck?" Due to his ability to walk and hold his hands up to his head he was assured at the moment it appeared he did not have spinal damage. However, any movement of his head might paralyze him. The liquor made him forget that statement many times as he would answer questions with a nod or shake of his head.   Constant reminders had to be made even during the x-rays and cat scans.

The reports from the radiologist indicated no fractures or

displacements of the vertebra. Pain was diagnosed as muscle spasms. "Does that mean I didn't break my neck?" Even before the affirmative answer was given he started to bawl with joy, with his girlfriend giving him a careful hug. They left with the neck collar in place, with medications to help the spasms and pain.

****

A 7 year-old child discovered an ATV could be a dangerous weapon. His father got on the vehicle behind him to offer the child a chance to "drive" the machine. The thumb lever accelerator was fully depressed by the inexperienced kid causing the ATV to jump forward at a sudden full speed. Panic set in and the grip on that lever got tighter with the father trying to slap the child's hand off the handlebar. In a short distance there was a crash of metal, plastic, rubber, and even flesh and bones into the side of the garage.

Both were thrown clear and brought to the ER by ambulance. The deformity of the child's right elbow was impressive. However, except for scratches and abrasions, he did not seem badly hurt. The father had rib pain and a few scratches.

When asked if he still liked ATVs the youngster said, "They are neat and awesome!" He was ready to get up and go again. The father said he would have to wait a few more years, especially to get on a big one. "Can we get a small one?" "We will see", was the stock answer.

The upper arm bone was shattered at the elbow, plus the top of the lower arm bone was soft with chips of bone instead of the typical nice rounded head. A temporary cast was put on, preparatory to getting him to an orthopedic surgeon. Surgery and a long physical therapy period would be ahead for this ambitious youth. The father only had bruised ribs. As the boy was being wheeled out he turned and repeated thru the pain medicine, "Neat and awesome!" All his father could do was shake his head.

****

Almost all of her 285 pounds were involved when she landed on her right knee. It was predicted she must have shattered the patella (knee cap) because of the screaming and loud moaning chiming together, creating a melody of pain. She must have learned way back that normal groans and utterances were not enough to express that amount of pain.

With a good 20 pounds of fat surrounding that knee joint, palpation to feel an either solid or soft kneecap was impossible. The yelps and swinging fists from the patient were also a deterrent to try a good examination. An x-ray was the only answer.

The staff made bets about whether it was broken or not, after she left for radiology to get the proof. It turned out to be a tie, as half believed it was fractured followed by 1/4 not fractured, and 1/4 unsure. The big question was how could so much weight landing on a kneecap not cause damage unless the fat saved her day or the story was not accurate as told. She said she slipped on the last step and fell forward landing on her knee, hearing something that sounded like a "crunch".

The pain shot given in mid thigh with an extra long needle was starting to take effect in x-ray because the echoing noises of pain were decreasing. Instead of screams there were "Ooohhhhs" and instead of whines there were "Dammits".

The sounds emanating toward the ER suddenly became more clear and louder. She was being wheeled back to her room. The x-ray technician was pushing the cot with one hand and holding his other hand over his ear.

Soon the radiologist report was sent to the doctor who then got a big smile, while turning to announce he was right. No bone damage noted. When the patient was notified of the diagnosis all she could bellow was, "Impossible, Impossible".

She was discharged with rather generous doses of pain medication and a muscle relaxer to help the spasms bound to occur in her leg. As one nurse commented, "Hopefully, it might relax her voice muscles."

****

The screams were mainly for the current situation and the sobs and crying were for a possible future calamity. These came from a middle-aged man with a relatively close range shotgun blast wound to the groin area. His blue jeans were shredded to threads from just below the belt line and extended half way down his inner leg. The blood spatters were from head to toe. He was a mess even in the eyes of a veteran trauma team. The loud verbal screams and sobs and swear words did not improve the scene.

The deputy sheriff was right behind the ambulance cot coming into the ER. The question the patient was avoiding was, 'Who did it?' He bellowed, "I don't know, just give me something more for pain. It really, really hurts." The deputy said, "If it was done this close you must have known who did it. You could have counted the hairs in his nose. Who are you protecting?"

A scissors was barely needed to cut away the rest of his pants to expose all the damage. It was a miracle that only one pellet entered the scrotum and his vital blood vessels had all been missed by a fraction of an inch. When he was informed of the damage, or lack of it, the sobs turned to laughter as he called out gratifying phrases aimed at the failed attempt of the female. By this time a lot more morphine had been given which helped him to put all the facts together sensibly instead of screaming.

The preferred position the patient took on the bed was flat on his back with legs spread wide apart because he frantically did not want to look at his wounds. They included a six-inch wide swath of flesh, and muscle torn to pieces. The ripping extended to the rectum like an episiotomy during childbirth. The penis was not harmed.

Much later as night was turning to daylight it was found out the shooter was a female. He was referring to his ex-girlfriend. She had come over to his house on a pretext and called for him to come into the bedroom. As he walked in, she aimed low and pulled the trigger.

As we packed the dressings into the wounds he would not stop talking about everything that had happened the past 6 months with "my woman" and why she would do this. She had broken off the relationship a month ago and did not like the fact that he was dating another gal. "This new woman is not a serious girlfriend, just a date, so why would she be so jealous?"

Every once in a while during the two hour bandaging he would stop talking, take a deep breath, and calmly ask, "Are you sure my sex life hasn't been affected?" Each time he was assured everything appeared normal, he would then continue his saga of "my woman". Surgical procedures would be in his future before he again would become "normal" for any woman. But he would surely never be "normal" for his ex girlfriend.

****

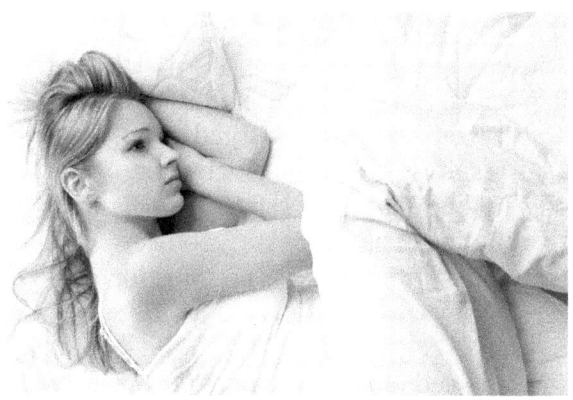

SPECIAL CASES

The most memorable patients are the ones a person will never forget. The ones who die are easy to list, of course, but the girl that "rises from the dead" (at least in her own mind) is unforgettable. Others are the devoted mother, the man living in extreme hardship due to improper medical attention, the wife who saved her husband, and the sweet blind gal, to name a few. These are the cream of the crop of memories.

****

A precious looking 11 year-old girl was brought in by ambulance from a significant auto accident. She was in a fetal position (curled in a ball) on the cot, and would not straighten out when transferred to the ER bed. There were numerous little glass cuts on her left shoulder and cheek. Her clothes had been cut away from her body to enable a good observation of any other injuries. Her breathing was normal, as were her other vital signs. The only unchanging symptom of her condition was her closed eyes and lack of reaction to verbal commands and requests.

Cat scans, x-rays, lab tests, and all other necessary tests were completed. She would allow her body to be moved to different positions for those tests, but would immediately curl back into the fetal position afterwards. Her eyes remained closed, sometimes, tightly closed. The situation was hard to deal with, because she didn't even cry when the stitches were done on the bigger glass cuts.

Most were thinking this was a brave girl, but the opposite was revealed.

Her parents, also brought in for treatment following the auto accident and ready to be discharged, were in the room crying over the lack of response from their daughter. A nurse knelt down beside the bed, moving just inches from the patient's face. With a low, quiet voice the nurse asked, "Are you dead?" One of the little girl's eyes did a slow little peek. The question was repeated even softer. Quietly, in the same quiet voice as the nurse, the child said, "I guess not."

The nurse stayed close and said, "Of course not, you are too pretty for us to allow anything bad to happen to you - and I was wondering - are you ready to go home?" Both eyes popped open and without moving her head she looked around. "Yes, you are alive and you can go home. "The girl smiled and proclaimed in a loud voice, "I have to go to the bathroom - bad!"

Laughter and joy filled the room, even after the patient was taken to the bathroom. She had been afraid she was either dead or going to die because no one had told her any different since the accident occurred.

After the bathroom run, the "newly reborn" girl stayed in the wheelchair as her mother presented her with a shopping bag. She peered inside, and saw it was a whole new set of clothes to wear since hers had been cut off during the initial treatment. Her mother had slipped out to buy them during the testing earlier that night. They were her favorite color and her eyes sparkled. She said she couldn't wait to change from the ugly hospital gown into a blue jump suit with a fur-collared jacket. Her bright and sincere smile was precious and contagious.

****

"This person is sick" was an obvious statement after one glance at the 46 year-old woman brought to ER by her husband. Unconscious, with eyes rolled upward, her skin color was ashen grey, her lips open and relaxed. Her breath sounds were slow and weak, but her heart was strong with very low blood pressure. The heart monitor activity was the only sign of life in the limp body, and her blood oxygen level was low to the point of being life threatening.

Her husband related her history of having been diagnosed with tongue cancer about 1 year ago. She had to live with a tube passed through her abdomen into her stomach to get food, water, and medications. Many surgeries were required for tube complications, and complications from the surgery on the tongue and throat. Just the day before, the surgeon had scheduled yet another surgery for an infection of the tube, which had become infected for the third time.

That evening, her husband had left her sitting in her chair while he made a trip to the store for groceries. When he returned, she was in the condition seen at present. There were scattered bottles of all her many medications around the chair, including some more from the bathroom medicine cabinet.

Some five hours later after numerous tests, she was somewhat stable with a breathing tube and ventilator. The highest substance found in her blood was rubbing alcohol, obviously poured thru her feeding tube. Her skin color never changed, the blood pressure stayed low, and she remained unconscious. She was put into ICU for monitoring. There were no changes until the third day, when her heart suddenly stopped. A "do not resuscitate" order had been signed by her husband and she presumably got her wish.

****

It was neither the medical problem nor how the treatment went that made this 45 year-old patient memorable. It was his attitude, in the midst of the terrible things that had happened to him in the past 6 years. He came into the ER with an extremely itchy rash all over his face, arms, hands, and chest. Upon assessment of the raised, almost blistering skin, a large scar on his mid abdomen was noticed. It sank deep, making star shaped wrinkles of scar tissue, with the focal point at the belly button.

During the treatment process, he was asked about that unusual scar on his abdomen. His nonchalant manner of answering minimized the event. He had gastric bypass surgery 6 years ago for an extreme overweight condition of 455 pounds. During the surgery something went wrong, and he went into a coma for 2 months. During that time, it was very hard to roll him due to his bulk and he got bedsores on his back and thighs. The scar on his abdomen was due to the stitches and staples continually being pulled open because of the pushing and pulling by staff to move him. He remained in the hospital for one year, and spent another 6 months in a nursing facility for rehab. Now weighing 190 pounds, he easily rolled over to show the other large scar on his rear.

When asked what he currently did for a living, he said, "Nothing, but not because I don't want to." Further explanation detailed his trials and tribulations. Due to brain damage his coordination was slightly skewed, and his speech was not perfect. No matter what the job consisted of, one of those skills was important. He could not find a job.

He lived on $500 per month with $300 going for rent. He watched television nearly 18 hours a day, but made sure he took a walk of at least 1 mile per day. He tried to mow lawns, but crashed the lawnmower into the house, due to "stupid moves". He kept looking for something he could do, and that occupied some of his time but always led to more rejections.

The question of a lawsuit was made, but even if he was able to afford the thousands of dollars to pursue a case, a win was not sure. If he did win even a million dollars all of it probably would be quickly spent on more treatments and hospitalizations, which then would nullify the Medicare that paid all of it now.

All the questions for this patient brought "matter of fact" answers with a smile. There was no evident depression, in mannerisms or words. In fact, he was cheerful and seemed to have accepted his fate in life, and would live it to the best. What a man! His gratitude for relief from the itchy rash was also sincere.

****

A sudden onset of sharp pain in the left chest was the complaint of a 39 year-old male as he stepped into the triage room. Since this single symptom alone does not mean a heart attack, more questions were asked, including medications or use of recreational drugs. He denied taking any kind of drugs, legal or illegal. He was placed in a cardiac work-up room with a monitor. Tests came back with slight signs of possible heart involvement.

He appeared cool, calm and collected about the possible diagnosis, and soon proclaimed all pain was gone after protocol medications. His concerns became obvious when he did not want to go home until he had answers as to the cause of the original pain. His wife was of the same conviction.

The cardiologist decided to do the angiogram, even if it was a borderline case for heart attack. The result was a moderate 80% blockage that was corrected with a balloon and stent. The blockage appeared smooth compared to normal plaque build-up, which is ragged – like an old sewer pipe. When he was put into a recovery room, he and his wife were again quizzed about their previous answer to recreational drug use.

His quick glance to his wife was a key sign. Methamphetamine use might be one cause of smooth blockage of arteries in the heart. If no drug use by this patient was actually the case, other tests had to be completed to learn the reason.

The man held his head low, and in a quiet shameful voice the truth was told. His wife stuttered, and finally said in a distinct voice, "Once in a while, we have used meth." They were assured the doctor/patient confidentiality was intact and he could probably go home in a day or so.

Remember to tell the truth – the whole truth, to your nurse.

****

The mother of the patient was amazing. She attended to her son's needs as no one else could. She had a routine that cycled every few minutes. She looked frail, but said she had been able to attend to him for years. That included putting him to bed, and getting him dressed.

He had advanced AIDS due to a blood transfusion 20 years before for his hemophiliac condition. During that time he became a paraplegic and lost his ability to speak. Four years ago his wife divorced him, because she could not deal with the advancing disabilities. Since then his mother had cared for him, along with friends and the community.

In the ER a temperature of 104 degrees made the skin of the 39 year-old man hot to the touch. Nasal congestion required nearly constant suctioning of his throat and nose. Four days earlier he had been diagnosed with pneumonia and had been taking liquid antibiotics and fever medications by way of his gastric feeding tube, inserted directly through the abdomen into the stomach. New IV antibiotics were started by infusion into his central line catheter.

While in the ER his mother was calmly, patiently and attentively attending to his every need including applying balm to his chapped lips; drying the sweat on his forehead; putting lotion on his hands and anything else she could think to do. Since he could not tell her his needs, she had to know by instinct what they were. She was a never-ending motion of caregiving , which made her "mother of the year".

When he was admitted upstairs to a room, the doctor said in his opinion this would be his last time to be admitted. In other words, he would not be going home from the hospital. The next day the prediction came true. The big question was, what would the mother do now?

****

Chest pain was the main complaint of a 33 year-old mentally challenged employee brought in from a local restaurant. In the time he had worked there, even with his handicaps, he had won the hearts of all the other employees. According to the boss who brought him to the ER the quiet, mild mannered dishwasher had never been late in three years. He worked past quitting time if asked and did his job with gusto, while humming or singing.

The report given was that he had completed all his work for the night and only then did he complain to fellow workers that most of the night he had been having "a hurt in my chest".

Noting he was sweating, they decided to have him checked out. The preliminary diagnosis was a stomach acid problem, quickly resolved by a special numbing drink called locally a "GI Cocktail".

A guilty look came over the patient's face when the cocktail worked and all pain was gone. In his normal quiet voice, the patient told his boss, "That special dish of the day looked good and I had it for my dinner. I didn't know it was going to do this." He did not fully understand why he had been on a "special diet" because of his "tender" stomach so when he saw this spicy food dish he decided to try it. A promise to "never do that again" was said with conviction.

The memorable part of this patient was not his illness or even his cure and final promise to watch what he ate. The patient had been in the ER for a total of 4 hours to rule out any heart, ulcer, or other problem that may have contributed to his chest pain. During this time, it was unbelievable the support shown by all his fellow workers. Besides the people present in the waiting room wanting to visit him, there were dozens of telephone calls of sincere concern for his well being. It was almost 2 AM before he was discharged and at least six people were still present to offer a ride home. The phone calls continued for another hour. It was touching how someone with a handicap that may have been cast aside was given a chance, and became the "mascot" of the whole team.

****

She was a hero to her family and her actions saved her husband's life. She was a slim, tiny lady with red hair and a good complexion for her 70+ years. She appeared to be a typical type "A" personality. Pride was written in her expression, but she tried to be humble.

Her 72 year-old husband had been asleep when he suddenly started to gurgle and grunt, then snore, followed by silence. This was not unusual because often he would snort, roll over off his back and continue sleeping.

She said she waited almost a minute and heard no sound. She nudged him, no response. She turned on the light and saw he was facing the ceiling with closed eyes, open mouth, and not breathing. She screamed for her daughter to call 911.

Nitroglycerin pills were on her nightstand, so she took one and grabbed his face to insert it under his tongue. It was difficult to accomplish, but she finally got it into place on the third try. In her mind, if one pill was good, then two would be better. This time insertion was no easier a task for her. In an excited state of mind, she was roughly manhandling his head to accomplish the mission.

Her daughter said she came into the room and witnessed her mother hollering at him and hitting him in the chest, stomach, and wherever her fist happened to land. She said there was a grunt, then a sneeze, and a projectile vomit as he started to sit up in bed.

EMS found him groggy and confused, but by the time they arrived at the ER the patient was alert. Standard protocol tests and exams did not find any unexpected results but he was admitted for observation as a precaution.

His wife was told she was a "HERO" in every sense of the word, even though the nitroglycerin pills had expired 3 years ago.

****

A young man of 13 years fell while running, landing on his face against a concrete block on the ground. He did not lose consciousness but his nose and forehead looked like a pizza with a ball in the middle. He had been quiet, except for his cries when the torn skin was scrubbed and stitches were placed.

Long after the repairs he remained still in bed, and only whimpered a weak answer to direct questions with both eyes closed. His mother was asked what his favorite treat might be. "A Big Mac," she replied. The nurse said, "Since we all know he isn't going to die if this young man can sit up and drink a glass of water he will be able to get out of here and enjoy that Big Mac."

Watching closely, we noticed he reacted just a little, but soon relaxed back to his previous position. Another minute passed while everyone remained silent. He opened his eyes and slowly started to move his arms into a position to sit up.

Without moans, groans, or squints of pain he very slowly got up onto his elbows and in about 2 minutes he was able to sit up. Clearing his throat, he whispered, "I'm thirsty." Only then did he "painfully", using two hands, hold the glass of water and sip slowly on the straw.

More minutes passed, in which the slowly recovering teen was able to get back into this world. Shortly he asked, "When can I leave?"

The boy's strategy on the slow "recovery" from no response to full response is termed "saving face". Once he realized he was NOT going to die he could not SUDDENLY come out of it and admit he had thought he was going to die - it would not be cool. So slowly "recovering" would be the best way to "save face". And the way his face appeared, it needed lots of saving – pun intended.

****

"Looks over life" was the motto of this memorable patient. Over the past few years she had endured liposuction and breast augmentation, plus lots of dieting. In her 36 years it had been a constant battle of the bulge. Although she sported a good figure and carried only 120 pounds on her 5'6" frame, she looked very ill due to nausea and vomiting.

Two months before, she had been diagnosed as diabetic. A specialized diabetic diet plus some oral pills had kept her illness under control until this week. According to her the diabetic pills were also making her gain weight and adding fat, so she had stopped taking them a week before. This resulted in a high sugar count over 4 times normal.

The treatment was to admit her to ICU with an IV insulin drip to bring the 436 reading slowly down to normal. She was asked why she would endanger her life over a few pounds that could be adjusted for with exercise and diet. Her lips tightened into a disgusted frown as her eyebrows lowered over her pretty brown eyes. Through clenched teeth she forcefully let everyone know, 'I have worked too hard to look good, and will not have it all ruined by a pill." In other words she was choosing "looks over life". Now was not the time to argue with her.

****

It was 5AM when a frequent ER flyer was noticed walking across the parking lot carrying a large envelope. His normal sob story involved pain of some part of the body requiring a narcotic pain shot. Seeing his left arm in a cast made everyone suspicious of something fishy.

As expected, this mid -30's man had a distinct high-pitched whine including a simple "Hello". This was going to be a good show for the slowest part of the night. He explained in a pseudo-convincing way how much pain he was in as he handed the envelope to the nurse. Each move of any part of the body, even his foot, produced a frown and grunt simulating pain in his injured arm.

The package contained an x-ray of his left arm showing a simple non-displaced crack of the smaller forearm bone. A simple touch by the doctor on the fiberglass cast brought another grunt, followed by a muffled yelp like a cat with a stepped-on tail. The reactions were well beyond the norm for a six foot 230 pound well built man. Continuous discomfort at rest with pangs of "severe pain" to the point of being unable to sleep was his best explanation.

Since no one had accompanied him to the hospital, protocol was no narcotic medication shot could be administered without a driver to take him home. He claimed his wife was in the car waiting for him. Why then, had he walked across the parking lot when the normal action would be for the driver to drop him off at the door and then go park the car? He was told we had caught him at that lie, and asked whether the pain was also a lie, which he denied.

The next ploy was to call his wife to come get him. That would be ok, but she had to be present inside the ER before the shot for his "pain" would be given. It was intriguing how much he was willing to do to get a fix. A half hour later she arrived, and he was discharged shortly after the narcotic shot. He was escorted by security to her car. The car was watched to make sure they were really leaving. We were not going to allow him to "pull" anything over on the system.

It was also shift change with nurses arriving. A few minutes later, one nurse came in saying she recognized a frequent flyer in the parking lot. She continued by saying he was getting out of one car and then getting into another car. Soon both drove out of the parking lot. She wanted to know what that was all about. The only answer was, "We've been had."

****

"This was one of the most peaceful passings I have ever had the privilege to witness," were the words the pastor spoke to the family of an elderly lady who had just passed away. She had been brought in by ambulance from a nursing home suffering "respiratory distress". Other complications listed in her medical history included renal failure with dialysis three times per week, Addison's disease, congestive heart failure, and high blood pressure, to name just a few.

The frail, unresponsive 81 year-old was placed in the trauma room emitting 'Niagara Falls' gurgles created by her inhalations in irregular and struggling efforts. Her mouth did not purse on exhalation, and her skin was cold, with fingers and lips a deep, dark, dull blue color. An IV was precariously placed through onion paper-like skin into a deep blue vein. The oxygen saturation meter was unable to pick up any reading.

Her family arrived shortly afterward, and was in the room when a DNR (do not resuscitate) paper from the nursing home was handed to the doctor. He told everyone to stand still and listen as he read the wishes of this lady. No CPR, no medications, nor any extraordinary methods were to be used to sustain life if her heart should stop beating, or her breathing should stop. She already looked peaceful, with her eyes open, looking upward to heaven. The family's pastor bent over to her ear and whispered, "Do you see a beautiful light? It is OK, you can go to that light." She immediately closed her eyes with a slight squint.

No one left the room or said a word. The crying baby in the next room also became quiet. All eyes followed the heart monitor for five minutes as the rate count went from 100 to 70 to 50 to 40 to 30, and then from just a squiggle to a straight line. Slowly, without a sound, everyone except the family and the pastor left the room. It was then he uttered the memorable words about the "most peaceful passing". What an experience to witness.

****

A good looking, husky black man entered triage complaining of severe big toe pain and a history of sickle cell, a common occurrence for this race. His cries of pain sounded like a howling wolf, and were heard in all corners of the ER. He was quickly admitted to a treatment room, along with the doctor and nurse.

A large amount of narcotic pain med was given by IV, after a blood draw to check the extent of the sickle cells. During the half hour the lab results were being run, the patient disappeared from the ER.

An investigation told us a fake name and address had been given, and a few calls to other local hospitals revealed similar happenings in the past few days. Our conclusion was a drug seeker had found a way to get a fix. We were onto him. He would be best off not to attempt that again in our ER.

****

Legally, she was blind since birth, but don't tell her that. This 20 year-old gal said she could see light and motion, so the word blind did not apply. Her mother said she was tested as being below average IQ, a fact put into doubt by the staff that cared for her.

A sweet sexy, and sincere voice was her biggest asset. Each time a person entered the room she would "see" the movement and ask, "Who is that?" The answer would be, "(Sally), your nurse." In an excited tone full of great enthusiasm, the patient would say, "Hello, Sally, my name is 'Julie!' It was so electrifying some would leave the room and come back in, just to hear the exuberant greeting again.

Two years before, the patient suffered an acute first- time seizure of unknown cause or origin. Her medication had been reduced gradually, since there had been no further incidences. She had been free of the medication for 2 weeks, when she had a grand mal seizure. The doctor explained to her the medicine had to be started again. And, yes, the side effects of hallucinations would return.

When she was told this, she "looked" at her mother straight on, and said with conviction, "I knew that was going to happen. Anyway, I kind of miss all those friends I had met and played with."

With a sweet, soft look, in a whisper her mother could not hear, she turned to her doctor and said, "They say there can be hallucinations, so if I act a little funny and even crazy at times, they blame the medicine when really I am just having fun." There was more IQ in that head then most would believe.

****

The red phone, a direct connection to the ambulance dispatch, rang only once before it was answered, "ER here". Dispatch: "This is a heads up, our ambulance is in route to a call of a person with a self-inflicted gunshot to the head." This was what the real ER was all about. The hairs stiffened on the back of the neck, the face flushed with the adrenalin rush, and protocol procedures flew through each well-trained mind.

Soon the ambulance report was being called into the ER. "We are coming to the ER with a conscious and alert 46 year-old male" – (With a gunshot wound?) – "blood pressure of 136 over 78 and a pulse of 100."

(What about the gunshot?) "He has a 1/4 inch wound near his left eyebrow with bleeding under control at this time." (Was it caused by a gunshot?) "Our arrival is about 5 minutes." (Is that all?)

The actual story: He was a paraplegic in a wheelchair staying in a local motel, and just had a quarrel with his girlfriend, who had stomped out of the room. The patient at this point said he didn't remember anything, but was guessing, "I must have passed out and fell, hitting my head against the bedside table. I don't know how long it was, but I do remember waking up on the floor realizing I was bleeding from somewhere. After getting back into the

wheelchair, I quickly went outside to get help because there was no phone in the room.

"The wheelchair did not stop, and tumbled off the curb spilling me onto the parking lot. It kept going down the hill, and I was just lying there. I couldn't get anyone's attention so I took my Derringer out of my pocket and fired both shots in the air to get help."

The first Good Samaritan arrived and saw a gun, with blood coming from a "wound" on the head. Of course he called 911 and reported a gunshot victim.

In the ER the wound was closed with super glue, and the patient was discharged to the care of his girlfriend. She had arrived shortly after the ambulance, also thinking that he had shot himself as reported to her by the police. She was crying hysterically with regret over their previous quarrelling. His final comment, "There must be a better way to win an argument."

****

He was curious, he was inquisitive, he was brave. This described the 5 year-old boy who had a large laceration just below his right knee. The first question he had, "Who is going to fix my "booboo?" He was told it would be a doctor. The nurse, with a mischievous smile, advised the boy that maybe he should ask the doctor, 'Are you good?' He did just that and got the answer, "Excellent", from the doctor. In a puffed chest position the curious lad said, "You better because I am going to watch you."

When he got to the treatment room the inquisitive boy was asked if he knew what was going to happen. His reply was that his brother, who had a booboo last year, told him exactly what was going to happen. "They are going to stick a huge needle right into the booboo and make it feel better. Then they are going to stick it again and again with a string until it is fixed." He was assured that was correct.

The doctor turned toward the counter with his back to the bed in order to draw up the numbing medication in the syringe, while the nurse was adjusting the large overherd light onto the "booboo". "What's that big light used for?" With a menacing smile, the nurse replied it was needed because doctors can't see very well.

When the doctor turned with the syringe in hand, the well-informed patient boldly pointed to the right knee and said, "It's right there!" The numbing procedure had to be halted for a while until the laughter got under control.

The rest of the procedure went without incident, and only a muffled cry was uttered when the "big needle into the booboo" was done. The rest of the process included the doctor answering a dozen questions while the stitching was completed. An extra large and impressive dressing was wrapped around the knee.

The patient left with a sincere 'thank-you for fixing my booboo, to each one involved. He added a comment to the doctor, "That nurse is wrong, I think you can see good!"

****

End stage liver failure plus kidney failure was the curse of a 49 year-old man. He was bloating and swelling like a balloon. 300 pounds on a small frame makes the situation hard to comprehend. He had been an alcoholic for many years and developed cirrhosis of the liver, helped only with comfort medications like narcotics.

He was quiet, pensive, and seemed to never look up but just stared down to his huge belly. When asked about pain he said it was not bad, but the grimacing told another story. His wife was present and remained silent, unless questioned directly.

In the past he had refused to sign a DNR (do not resuscitate) paper, hoping for a chance to survive this disease. This night he, his wife, and the doctor knew he had very little time left on this earth. His breath sounds were weak, and the monitor indicated his heart was only pumping little ripples of blood into the veins instead of a beat. The only pulse able to be palpated was in his neck and upper left arm. It was a struggle for him to continue into the next minute but determination kept him going.

When shown the DNR papers this time, he just kept looking at them without comment for many minutes. Then with a nod of his head, he reached his hand out for the pen. As he pressed the point of the pen to the paper, tears started down his face, and that of his wife. She hugged his neck and he kept writing. By the time he finished the unreadable scribbles of his name he was actually bawling out loud. It was the greatest effort he had completed since arrival. A teardrop landed on his signature to seal the act.

He was admitted to a private room with orders for as much comfort meds as needed. About 3 hours later word was sent down to the ER he had passed away. It was a heart-wrenching event.

****

The End

www.ingramcontent.com/pod-product-compliance
Lightning Source LLC
Chambersburg PA
CBHW072024190526
45166CB00015B/332